Weight Loss Interviews: The Real Life Stories Of How 13 People Lost Weight In Their Own Unique Way

Dr. Howard Rankin

COPYRIGHT NOTICE

COPYRIGHT © 2014 by Talent Writers ALL RIGHTS RESERVED. No part of this publication is allowed to be reproduced in any form without written permission from the author. Only reviewers are allowed to quote brief passages from this publication.

Brenda Johnston

Results Not Guaranteed, They're Earned!

I was super skinny growing up. I lived in a small town in Canada until I was ten years old. Mom cooked healthy meals, for the most part, and I was always running around outside -- and even inside.

When I was ten, my parents felt I needed better educational and life opportunities, and we moved to a much larger town just outside of Toronto -- Whitby. I was active, involved, didn't have a problem and mom was still cooking for me.

Then I went to college. I weighed about 165 and was 5'9". Initially, I commuted to the International Academy of Design where I was studying marketing and design, then finally moved out to be on my own. Now I had unlimited access to all of those foods I had been deprived of, or thought I was. I went nuts. I was doing the college thing -- drinking, eating, and having fun. I put on fifteen pounds -- and that's when I was still living at home. I finally moved out when I was 21. I was now two hours away from my parents. Finally, independence! Awesome! But I didn't know how to cook! OMG! I'm going to eat Mr. Noodle and Kraft dinners every day.

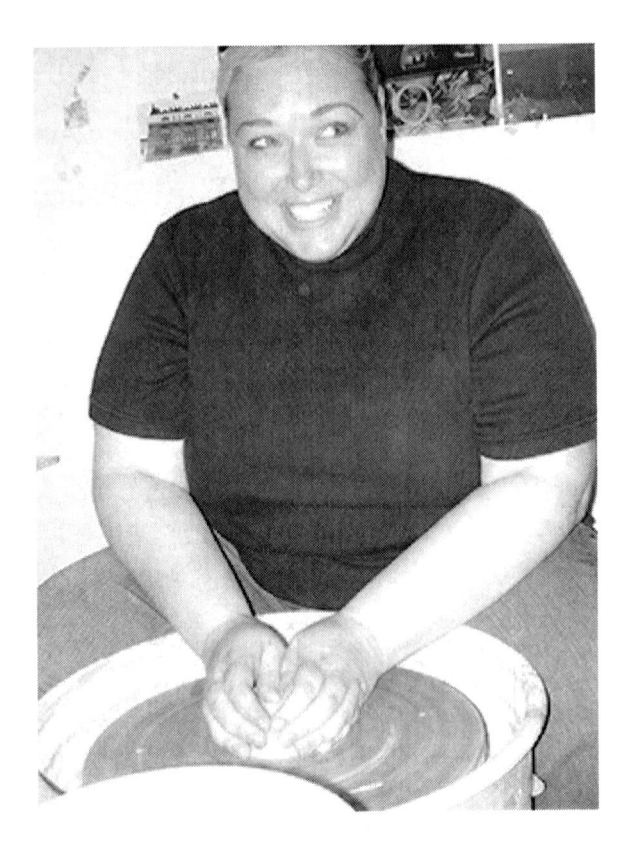

I soon landed my first advertising design/ marketing job. It was stressful, crazy deadlines and of course, my first job and I didn't want to screw up. My solution was to not eat much during the day but drink four very large Snapples; water was boring, and the Snapples seemed to keep me full. At the time, I didn't realize they were full of chemicals. Why would I? No one teaches you that. So, I went from being fairly active- to sitting on my butt- drinking sugar water all day long. I was working long, weird hours, not eating very well and being fairly stressed.

The weight started to creep on. I didn't think about it much -- or at all. I was 180. I continued that trend. I've had an underactive thyroid since the age of 15, so I started to blame my weight gain on that. Then, I blamed my weight gain on the washer/dryer in my apartment complex. For some strange reason, the washer and dryer kept shrinking my clothes. But the scale also said I was now over 200 pounds. Well, that's okay because I won't get to 225. Or 240. Or 250.

By this point I had stopped getting on the scale, likely because the one I had, only went up to 240lbs.

I could see that I was getting bigger but no one said anything. Well, that's not quite true. My parents did notice that I had gained "a little bit of weight." They actually shelled out a little money for me to go to Weight Watchers. Over the next several years, I went back to Weight Watchers over 11 times, meaning I literally signed up 11 different times for new sessions, thinking I would have a different result. Each time, however, I had the same result -- no real, as in maintained, 'weight loss, changed my life,' success. I know Weight Watchers works for a lot of people; it just wasn't working for me, probably because I wasn't ready to make it work.

By now, I was 24, and I had just gotten married. I weighed 232. I resolved to come back from my wedding and really do something about this weight. I did not want to get any heavier than 232, period.

So, a few months later, I was reading about Dr. Bernstein's program, a very low-carb diet designed to control blood-sugar levels. I signed up for a lot more than "a little bit of money," with the expectation that I could lose the excess weight in no time at all. I was on it for six weeks, about 800 calories a day, and not exercising (fortunately, given that I was on 800 calories a day). I lost fifty pounds in the first month. But, I didn't look good. I looked gaunt and unhealthy. My skin color even changed, and my hair had lost its shine, but that didn't matter because the scale was going down, and in my head, that was ALL that mattered.

While on the program I happened to mention to one of the nurses, I was hungry a lot of the time. Duh! The nurse gave me the solution.

"Go to the store and get a supply of flavored fizzy waters. The bubbles in those drinks will help fill you up." Well, who am I to argue with a trained health professional? I did just what she said.

It didn't work very well. I started to get severe stomach cramps, largely due to the fact, that I am sensitive to aspartame. The filling fizzy waters were full of that, along with about a zillion other chemicals. But again, how was I supposed to know that? For the longest time, I had a diet coke addiction, drinking at least three a day. I didn't drink coffee or tea, and the diet soda was one way to get caffeine. Looking back, that sounds disgusting, but it was my habit for a long time. Incidentally, I can tell very quickly -- like 3.2 seconds -- whether a food has aspartame in it. I bloat like mad and get a crazy headache.

I kept the Bernstein weight off for about two months. I went back to tell them I wanted to go on maintenance and onto a more moderate program. The doctor responded very compassionately. He said: "Well, if you want to be fat for the rest of your life, you can go on maintenance now." I remember thinking "I'll show you!" then I stopped at McDonald's on the way home and ate three hash browns, a sausage and Egg McMuffin. Take that!!

I considered the various forms of bariatric surgery but, fortunately, the idea of surgery scares the heck out of me, so it was never really an option. And looking back now, after maintaining a 145-pound weight loss for several years, I am so glad I didn't go that route. It has worked for some people that I know, but it's just not for me. What that surgery does, in my humble opinion, is buy you some time where it is easier to change your eating and exercise habits. But, if you don't make that change there's a very real risk you'll regain all your weight back -- and then some.

Of course, I eventually regained the Bernstein weight loss and added some more for good measure. In fact, after losing the 50 pounds in those first few weeks, I gained about 100 over the course of the next four years. That was okay because at that point, I decided that I was indeed meant to be the funny, big and curvy girl. And 315 pounds.

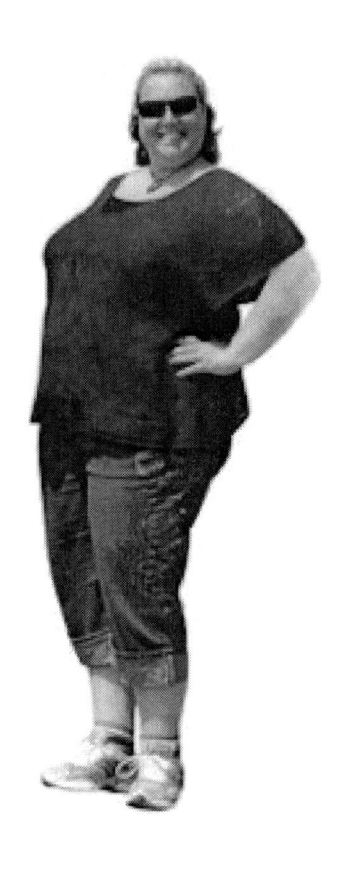

Along the way, I tried a few programs like Herbal Magic, Atkins, Weight Watchers, the Cabbage Soup Diet, pretty much every diet known to mankind, and possibly a few other species, too. At one point, I sat down and calculated how much I had spent on weight-loss programs. It wasn't a little bit of money. It was close to $15,000 - 20,000. That's a conversion rate of about $130 for every pound gained.

I was working in marketing, and some of our clients were in the health and diet industries, so I was reading a lot about the latest products, and buying into most of them. Not that it was really helping. On my 30th birthday, my husband at the time and my parents threw a giant party for me. Afterwards, I saw the pictures of the party, and I didn't like what I saw. In fact, my reaction to the photos of me was, "Who the hell is that obese girl?" I remember staring at those pictures and crying secretly and then throwing them away. I resolved, right there and then, that it was time to take action. Now I had hit the landmark birthday, I needed to get control of my life and my weight. This had gone on for too long. The time was now. I was ready!

Three years went by, and nothing happened. Well, things happened but they weren't anything to do with my taking control of my weight, health or my life.

When I was 33, my husband and I had gotten an invitation to go to a wedding that was on a cruise ship. "Oh my God, I don't want to be the fat girl on a cruise ship."

Even so, the self-deception and rationalizations continued. I was starting to have pain and discomfort in my back and joints and was convinced that it was because the mattress was getting old.

Fortunately, the insurance company that I now worked for had a fitness center, and I decided to ask the fitness coordinator for recommendations for a personal trainer. I knew at this point that exercise was the way to my salvation. In my youth, I was very active. I was into dance -- some jazz, some tap -- played volleyball, soccer and would also go the gym. Back then, I always assumed I was going to stay skinny. It never crossed my mind that one day I would weigh over 300 pounds.

I duly met with the sports trainer whom the fitness coordinator had recommended. Being a 'Go Big or Go Home' sort of gal, I chose the best trainer because, after all, having the best trainer will make it all that much easier, right?

So, the trainer looked me and asked me when I wanted to start. I said, "Maybe in a couple of weeks. I need to get the money together, get myself prepared."

"Okay," said the trainer, "I'll see you here first thing in the morning. We'll work out a payment plan."

I started going into the gym before work. I would actually be at the gym by 7:30 -- and I lived forty-five minutes away. I saw him three times a week. And weak was how I felt after the first few days. To be more precise, I thought I was going to die. My muscles were so unconditioned I couldn't do a basic sit-up, something that was easy for me in my youth. My gut was in the way. That was a huge moment, the moment when I seriously asked myself, barely holding back the tears, 'What have you done to yourself?'

But I got through it and continued to work out like crazy. At the end of the first month, I got on the scale and discovered that I had lost -- five pounds. What the hell?

"You're down five pounds but your body fat is down a lot more than that," the trainer told me. I started to understand the difference between weight and body fat.

Working out hard for the year, I lost 54 pounds. That didn't seem like a lot to me but the fact was that my body fat percentage had gone from nearly 60% to 49%. I was still half fat, but it was going down.

At this point, I wasn't eating badly but I still hadn't learned how to eat well. I was watching TV one day and a woman was on it and her name was Tosca Reno. She was talking about healthy eating. I was so impressed I went straight out and bought her *Eat Clean Diet* book. I thought it was a diet -- as in 'weight loss' -- book, but soon discovered that her book was about eating clean for life. That book literally changed my life.

I started to learn about sugar, fats and healthy fats and all sorts of mind-blowing things. Actually, after doing the Dr. Bernstein 'program' I got my Nutrition and Wellness Specialist Certification. Now, I was going to instantly be an expert, and it would transform me into a healthy eater. It didn't, of course, but the certificate was nice. If the certificate itself was still rolled up in a drawer somewhere, its main benefit would soon unfold.

As my health and weight loss journey started to roll, it occurred that I could do some work-site wellness. In fact, not wanting to waste momentum, I approached my company with the idea of staging a weight loss competition for the employees. The idea stemmed from the fact that I saw employees coming to the gym every morning and weighing themselves. It was also the time when the Biggest Loser was making a big splash and as a marketer, I knew how to jump on a bandwagon.

My company bought into the idea. We charged each participant in the 12-week course $10, and that went into the prize money pot. We anticipated we would have about 40 participants. I put together a little brochure and was scheduled to announce the program in one of our meeting rooms.

I remember standing at the front of the meeting room and looking over my notes. I like notes; I like to be prepared and know exactly what I am going to say. I looked up and saw that the room was overflowing with people. There was no room for all those who wanted to get in!

It was at that moment; I put down the notes I had written. I took a deep breath, and I just talked. I just decided to tell my story. It was the first time that I had really let the walls down in public. I totally felt naked. I told them about my denial. The clever rationalizations, the frustration and the disgust. When it was over, I felt that a huge weight was lifted off me in some strange way. It might have been psychological weight rather than fat, but it was just as important, if not more so.

By the time I got back to my desk, I had over 40 e-mails from people who had directly or indirectly heard me talking about my story. They appreciated my honesty. They appreciated the fact that I had shared my struggles. They appreciated the fact that this was a real story with real results. It wasn't edited or photo-shopped.

That was a turning point for me. I put it all out there, with honesty, and got a lot of love in return. No fat girl jokes, no cynicism -- just warmth and appreciation. Perhaps it's okay to be honest; I mean really honest, and not just with others, I mean with yourself, that moment, I became a much better person. Prior to that, been a glass half-empty person, often in victim mode. Now, beginning to become much more positive, even spiritual.

My view of life changed. I became more grateful. I appreciated life more, the seemingly small details, and the people. I'm a completely different person, now. I am grateful for my health, for my friends, for everything. I used to see limitations, but now I only see possibilities. I'm a huge believer in the power of positive affirmations. I happened to get mine tattooed on me, extreme perhaps and my Mom hates it, but they remind me how far I have come and what is possible. When I lost my first twenty pounds and kept it off, I got the word "believe" tattooed across my wrist in Tibetan Sanskrit. When I lost the 145lbs and kept it off for two years, I had the words "mens sana in corpore sano" tattooed across my forearm. It means "a healthy mind in a healthy body." I'm working on a new one, it says "Limitless," because that's what life is about, limitless possibilities.

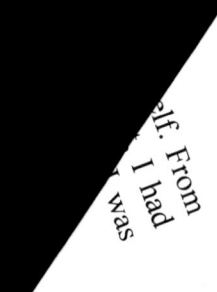

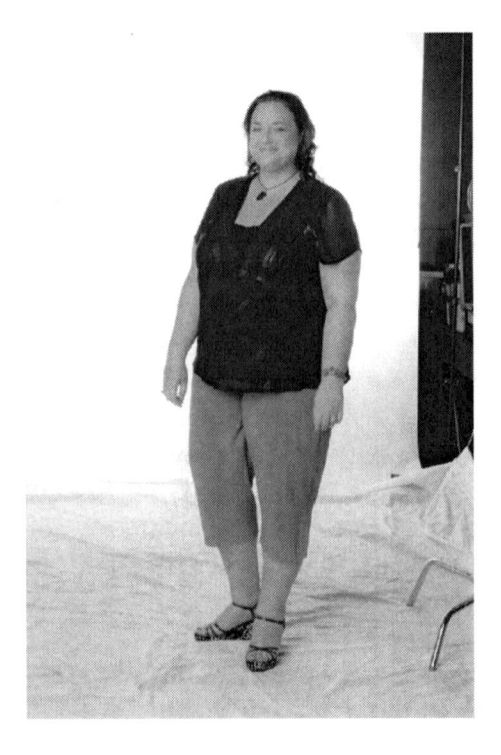

Letting go of the ego is huge, and talking to the people in that room was the start of letting go. My eyes were opened as much as anyone else's that lunchtime.

Part of my former negativity came- I'm sure- because of poor nutrition and lack of exercise, which have a very negative effect on your brain. Now, if I miss a day exercising, or don't eat too well, I'm cranky. My energy is low and my mood not so good. But, all that was in the past when I suggested starting the work-site weight loss challenge.

There are 800 employees in my work-site building. 180 people signed up for the program, and the company was so impressed they donated extra money to increase the prize money to $1000. I was also able to get donations for even more prizes from local businesses. Over 12 weeks those 180 people lost a total of 800 pounds.

Before long, there were people coming into the gym in the morning wanting to meet with me, and work out alongside me. Around this time, I also decided that a lunchtime workout would be fun, not in the gym but simply exercising outdoors. I designed an outside lunchtime group class that used the natural landscape, benches, curbs, as "equipment." The idea caught on. People at my work started to e-mail me and ask if they could join in. At one point, I had twenty-five people participating. These lunch workouts were almost daily, and soon I discovered that people who were fit wanted to join in, too, which at the time, blew my mind a bit.

Working for an insurance company, it wasn't long before it occurred to me that if anyone got hurt on these lunchtime jaunts, I might get sued. I decided it would be a good idea to get my physical fitness trainer certification. And, of course, I didn't want just any certification, I wanted to get the best one available.

I studied hard for six months, took the exam -- and failed. I tried twice more before finally getting certified. Part of the problem was that there was a lot of math and science and I'm an Arts girl. I subsequently got certified in teaching spinning classes, and in various other equipment-based activities like the TRX suspension system.

Now I was certified; people asked me whether they could pay me to train them. A fledgling business was born.

The organization which certified me as a Nutrition and Wellness Specialist, CAN-FIT PRO, staged regular events, and as a graduate of one of their courses, I soon got notice that Tosca Reno was going to appear at an upcoming event. I was determined to go and meet her. I took along my tattered copy of her book, replete with sticky notes about things I had found useful and even a photo of me at my heaviest.

I did get to meet her. As I gave her my book to sign, the "fat Brenda" photo (as I call her) dropped out. "Is this you?" the authoress asked somewhat incredulously. At this point, I was down about 80 pounds, but I looked completely different.

"That's amazing," she said. She promptly called one of her colleagues over and asked me whether I would mind being featured on their clean eating website. Of course not!

I was indeed featured on her website in November. Soon, I got another call from Tosca's entourage, and they wanted to feature me in their magazine as a success story. The story was great, and it was nice to be recognized. But there were other consequences.

When I was featured on the *Eat Clean Diet* website and in *Clean Eating* magazine, the company proudly publicized my stories, and I soon felt like a minor celebrity.

As a result of this new-found fame, I now had 800 people watching me. Watching what I ate, when I worked out, frankly, when I did anything. I couldn't let them down.

By now, I was really doing well with my nutrition and exercise. But soon, disaster struck. I damaged my ankle and had to stop my routine. That was scary. There was part of me that felt I would wake up tomorrow and weigh 315 pounds again. But, that injury was a blessing in disguise.

Blessings in disguise. I really believe that everything happens for a reason. Not necessarily that there's some mystical force pulling the strings of your life but rather that events present you with an ever-changing set of opportunities. Whatever happens, there are now new challenges. If you embrace them, you will grow in ways you never thought likely. You have to put in the work; you have to take the responsibility, but when you do, you will know that whatever happens is another step in your destiny.

So, now that my exercise was severely curtailed I had a new appreciation of the importance of nutrition. I was terrified of putting weight back on which meant that I had to be especially vigilant about what I put in my mouth. I really became fascinated with food. I researched more. I was eating really clean; no fried or processed food, minimal sugar and a lot of fruits and vegetables.

When I was able to get back into my exercise regime, I now had both parts of the equation -- the food and the exercise -- working in harmony.

My body started to change amazingly. In photos of that time, it appears that I am going along losing weight and then, around this time, I really look different.

I started entering races, something I NEVER imagined I would have the guts to do, including the Men's Health Urbanathlon in Chicago. I may not have been the fastest person or the strongest, that wasn't the point. I was just proud of myself for completing the events. I wanted to test my body, to see how far I could take it. After about six months of working out, it honestly stopped being about vanity and became about how far I could push myself.

Given my highest weight and terrible lifestyle habits, I should have had hypertension and diabetes and a host of other problems, but I didn't, and I wanted to fix it, so I never would. I did have high cholesterol and was on some medication, and my blood pressure was high but not horrible; my resting heart rate was 85 when I was at my highest weight. Now, it's normally between 49-55, which is a huge difference. People need to remember it's not just about the changes people can see; it's about the changes on the inside too.

I remember visiting my doctor. She's a really tiny woman and there was a poster on the wall behind her, which said, "Ask me about healthy weight loss options." So I did. "Get off your butt and start moving," was her medical opinion.

I now wanted to see if I could build muscle. About a year ago, I got into lifting weights, like serious lifting, to see how it could shape my body and learn first-hand the role these exercises have in fat reduction. In case you're wondering the answer is that it has a huge difference. For example, after I lost my 145 pounds, people kept asking me where my skin went. I told them it was still there, where it was meant to be. Losing the weight slowly and using resistance exercises, spared me sagging skin. I have a stretch mark or two but nothing that needs surgery, which is good because remember I told you already, surgery is scary to me.

I also decided to go back to school to get a two-year certification in advanced holistic natural nutrition. Of course, I wasn't doing much else except my full-time job, working out intensely, helping some clients with their own fitness goals and others with nutrition, and running lunchtime work-outs.

As much as I love training with people, what I am most passionate about is nutrition.

People don't understand that they're eating themselves to death. Poor nutrition contributes significantly to virtually all the major diseases. Being in marketing, I've worked with companies that have promoted unhealthy products that are touted as healthy choices or added healthy benefits. I think it's my cosmic duty to make up for any harm I've indirectly caused by helping promote unhealthy stuff.

Unfortunately, the fact is that not enough people realize the critical role of nutrition. We're all far too consumed with convenience and changing how you eat isn't convenient.

I weigh and measure everything. Despite what I've heard some of my colleagues say, it is crucial to count calories. It has educational value and promotes awareness, without which you cannot change. Many people are, contrary to popular opinion, not eating enough. When I think about how I used to eat, I think of myself as an anorexic fat person. For example, I was severely restricting fat intake to no more than 20 grams a day. It's the quality of calories that matter! I can eat 2700 quality calories a day today and not gain weight because of the type of calories I'm eating and the level of activity that I have.

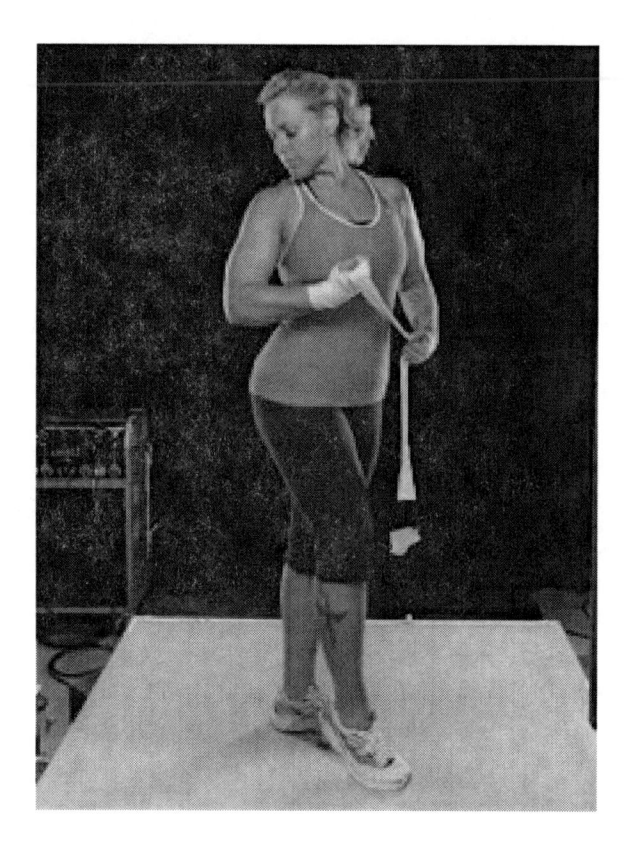

Part of the problem is information overload. There's too much information, too much conflicting information, too much nonsense. No wonder people don't know what to do. That's why I love helping them sort it out and individualizing their own plans. Oh, in case you didn't know, "natural" flavors are made by frickin' scientists.

I eat six times a day. Yep, six times a day.

I get up at 5:30 and typically have toast, peanut butter and a protein shake.

After my workout at around 8am, I have something like a small omelet, fruit and toast.

At around 10:30, I typically have a snack of Greek yogurt with protein powder and/or a sweet potato and cottage cheese.

Lunch is some chicken or fish with rice or pasta or quinoa.

My 4pm mid-afternoon snack consists of vegetables, possibly Tilapia, Chili and/or a protein shake.

Dinner is typically chicken or fish, stir-fried with vegetables.

I try not to go more than four hours without food. I have a lot of protein because it keeps me full. Often people think of their proteins last, rather than first.

If I'm training for something specific, I eat carbs at night but otherwise usually only have those earlier in the day, especially the higher glycemic ones. It's when my body needs them the most.

I like to eat. One of my favorite treats is movie popcorn with butter -- maybe once every couple of months, or a glass of wine with a meal on the weekend. Some of my clients just don't want to give up the booze and to be honest it's tough to lose weight if you're drinking alcohol very regularly.

People allow setbacks to define them. I've been through a separation recently, and people were waiting for me to relapse. It's true; I did gain a few pounds, but I knew what I was doing and didn't let it get out of hand. I had a pity party, but it was short-lived. I was bothered though.

When I had to face getting back in the dating scene I was scared. It was a huge part of my journey. I was together with my husband for 18 years. I don't know how to date! I was horrified at the prospect that I would meet someone and they would find out I was fat, and they wouldn't want me anymore. Somebody was also eventually going to see me naked!! So, I put on some weight and used it as an excuse. My self-sabotaging thoughts and habits died hard. I was afraid of success. I mean, if you don't succeed, you can't fail, right?

This sort of thinking has dogged my life up until recently. My industry is a man-dominated field. So what did I think? I don't want to be successful because I am pretty, but because I am smart and driven. I'm sure that was one of the reasons -- or is that rationalization? -- That I gained weight. I would be successful despite my weight. But, when I was separated, I didn't want to hide behind a layer of fat. I needed a year to figure out who I was. Everything I thought I knew was now gone.

Our marriage had been struggling for a few years, and I was okay with it ending amicably. There were people who thought I left because I'd lost weight and thought I was all that; they had no idea what really went on. I needed to keep my head on straight and stay focused. The truth of the matter was we had simply grown into two very different people from when we first met. We got married at a young age. It's sad, but it happens. I've learned that it can take more guts to leave a situation that isn't working for you than to stay in it and be unhappy.

Initially, however, I wasn't ready to date. It was one of the most horrifying experiences of my life, especially the thought of online dating. The old thoughts started to appear. "I don't want some to like me just because I'm good looking." "Test them by making yourself less attractive." No, I'm not going back there. Stop! I told myself that I would meet the right person, so stop eating M and Ms. I actually did something that I had never done; I went out of town for the weekend by myself. I needed to experience independence, that my feelings and experiences, the whole transformation, was real. It was. I got more comfortable about the whole dating thing.

So, I have lost 145 pounds and kept if off for more than four years, now. Clearly, there are times when old habits want to emerge. Anyone who tells you they just disappear is flat out lying. That's one of the problems with the weight loss industry -- it's unrealistic. Too much hype. When I was on my journey I needed to see someone like me, not unrealistic Biggest Loser stories. It is possible. It's also work. As I say on my website, "Results not guaranteed, they are earned!"

Before   After

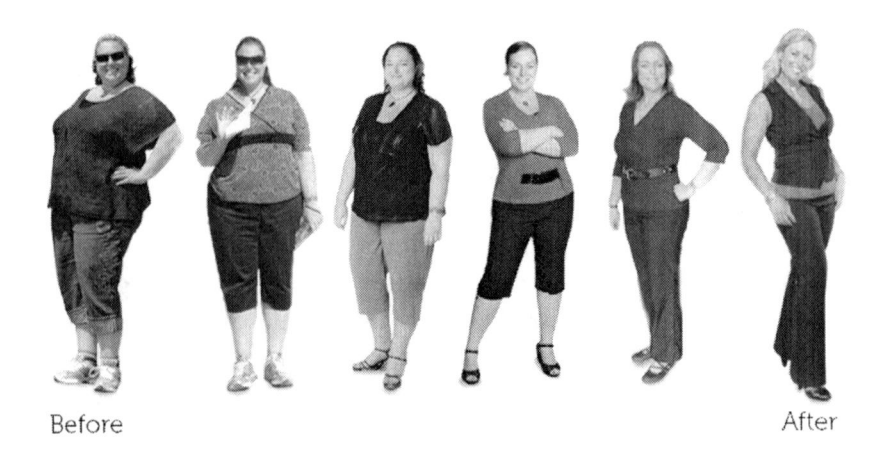

When those old thoughts and habits want to take over, I remind myself how far I've come. That conversation with myself is easier and easier to have. It might take me a few days to really get refocused, but it does happen.

When I'm not feeling so good about myself, I also get into one leg of my fat pants to remind myself of where I was. And talking of pants, often when I'm clothes shopping I find that I have taken the wrong size of, say, pants into the dressing room. I put one leg through, and I realize the clothes are way too big. In fact, it took me a long time to realize I didn't need to go to the heavy girl store any more.

When my resolve wants to take a vacation, I also look at my website and comments from people I have helped. And being a professional helper, I feel the need to be a good example and certainly not let anyone down. And it also helps that some people at work are very complementary and look at me as their role model.

Another reminder I use comes in the form of plastic replicas of a pound of fat and a pound of muscle that I have on my desk. It's a good conversation starter, and it motivates me.

I also make sure that I always have a goal. It's important that there's a more immediate goal than 'some day.' The goals I make aren't weight-loss goals, they are short-term objectives, like training for a race, or designing and implementing a 12- week fitness program.

Nobody tells you how to set goals. I do. It's important. Also, I hardly ever weigh myself or my clients. It's not about the scale. The measure I'm more interested in is body-fat percentage.

At first, when I lost the weight, my parents were cautious. They didn't realize initially about the total transformation. I know they're proud. I'm sure they were worried when I separated and were concerned, as several people were, that I would relapse.

I hope I've influenced my parents. They've changed the way they eat. Dad walks more -- and he needed to. He was diagnosed as diabetic and has since lost 80 pounds. Both of my parents are now more active. They travel and do some cool things, like snorkeling. I remember that when I was growing up, mom and her friends were always talking about the next diet or weight-loss program they were going to do. I grew up thinking that dieting was what everyone did, regardless of their weight.

I want to educate people about healthy living. It's simple, but it's not easy. Once you know what to look out for, you can make changes. I wish I could walk up to some people, grab them by the scruff of the neck, shake them and convince them that they can do it. It's not about weight loss it's about maintainable weight loss. You can't just lose weight and be fixed. It's a mind-body-spirit transformation.

For me, there's nothing greater than helping others transform their lives. I can get so excited about it that I have to remind myself to calm down! I realize that everyone has to have goals, and I teach people how to set the best realistic goals for them.

I train employees during lunch hours. In the evenings, I teach classes, where I typically have between 15 and 20 participants. I also do some training out of my house and virtual training internationally. I do clean eating coaching, and nutrition consults via Skype. I have clients all over Canada, the US, the UK, even as far afield as India.

I have recently created a 50 video course where I go into my story even more in depth. I the good, the bad and anything I learned along the way that may help you. They are available for free at www.inslim.com.

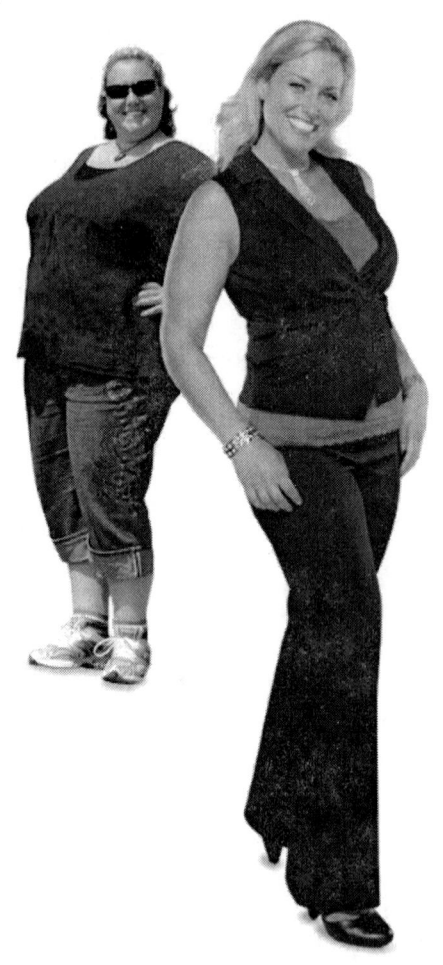

I have never been this focused in my life. It's falling into place. I know my life's purpose.

Do you know yours?

Don Whiting

In Need of Inspiration

When my brother and I were growing up in the Canadian Maritimes, we had all the advantages of my family's upward mobility into the middle class. We could have whatever we wanted and that meant unlimited junk food. We could dine out -- and dine out we did at KFC, McDonald's, and other fine eating establishments. Our cupboards were chock-full of chips, Twinkies and other fine foods. I thought this was the normal way to eat, what everyone did.

All of us were big, but again I thought this was normal. But, going to school was an eye-opener. I was the biggest kid in the class. I remember going to the doctor to get a permission slip for an upcoming Cub Scouts field trip. He gave me and my parents the permission slip and also a warning. I needed to watch my weight and go on a diet. My parents took the permission slip but not the advice. The weight piled on.

I was bullied a lot, especially in high school. I was taunted and teased. I was a lumbering fat kid who was easy to push around. It didn't help that I was a latchkey kid, too. I would go home, lock the door, escape to my video games and bury my sorrow in chips, snacks, and anything that would temporarily alleviate my depression. I was in a cycle, and it was vicious. It was keeping me trapped.

If truth be told, I was seriously depressed. But the truth never was told. I was too ashamed. I didn't think I would be taken seriously, so why bother. I thought about suicide but wasn't convinced I had a sure-fire way of being successful, and I would only end up making it worse. So the shame prevented me from saying anything, and I kept going back to the isolation of video games and Oreos. I have to say that as bad as it was, it was easier back then. I could come home and shut it all out, unlike today where the shame and taunting follows you 24/7 in the digital world.

One particularly cruel prank the bullies played on me was in 10th grade. The "cool kids" stole books and electronics from some other students and then put them in my locker. Then they "ratted me out" to the principal. I was duly called to the principal, who didn't believe that I had nothing to do with it and he threatened to call my parents.

"We know you did it," he insisted.

The worst thing about the whole incident was that I knew my parents -- at least my dad -- would side with the principal. I was terrified that the principal would call them. I pleaded my case.

He didn't believe me, but he didn't call my parents. He returned the stolen goods to their rightful owner, and that was that. That wasn't a terribly satisfactory outcome. Everyone thought I had done it, except the kids who pinned it on me, and they got away with it scot-free. I felt like I had nobody in my corner. From the domineering father, to the school administration, to my classmates – it seemed everyone was against me, and I felt very isolated. My best friend in the whole world was food.

My response to this hell was to dive into schoolwork and reconstruct my self-esteem through academic success. I was very successful, getting really great grades and in the process, of course, making myself even less popular, if that were possible.

Obviously, Gym was always my lowest grade. I hated it with a passion. The gym teacher would always give me a terrible grade, affecting my overall grade-point average. Of course, I deserved a terrible grade as I hardly did any physical activity. At one point, I played a little baseball, but I was always the last one to be picked because even if I hit the ball it would take me about an hour to get to first base -- or that's how it felt. I was destined to a sedentary life for sure.

So, I was generally isolated, although I did hang out with a few nerdy, geeky kids, who were similarly social outliers.

I never got on the scale at this time. I'm not sure where the scale was. But the taunting continued and led to more emotional eating. I guess I was about 180 and 5'6" in 11th grade.

I survived high school. That's how I really think of it. I was happy when it was over. At no point during the high school years did I even consider doing anything about my plight. I was focused on schoolwork and my grades, and I didn't even want to think about my weight. It was too painful. And when I did think about it, I had absolutely no confidence that I could lose it, or more accurately, keep it off.

This is very important. I'm a person who believes in data, thrives on information. Even in high school I had no reason to think that anyone could lose a significant amount of weight and keep it off. I saw no examples of that, and I had no one telling me it was possible.

I accepted a place at St Mary's University in Halifax to study computer science. I continued to live at home. But the change from high school to college made a difference. It was a fresh start. None of my high school tormentors would be there. Nobody knew my history. I made a concerted effort to be more sociable by getting involved in a number of clubs and activities like the Environmental Club and the school newspaper. I could contribute and being around like-minded people made socializing easier.

But my increase in social activities didn't improve my eating. I was eating on campus, which is generally not the healthiest place to eat. I was eating a lot of pizza and burgers.

I also had a part-time job working at Kmart selling shoes. On Friday afternoons, when I got paid, I would go to McDonald's and take advantage of their $1 cheeseburger promotions. I actually bought 20 cheeseburgers for $20 and ate them all during the course of the afternoon. I had earned the nickname "Jughead" from my friends.

There were also all-you-can-eat contests at Pizza Hut, and I won several of those!

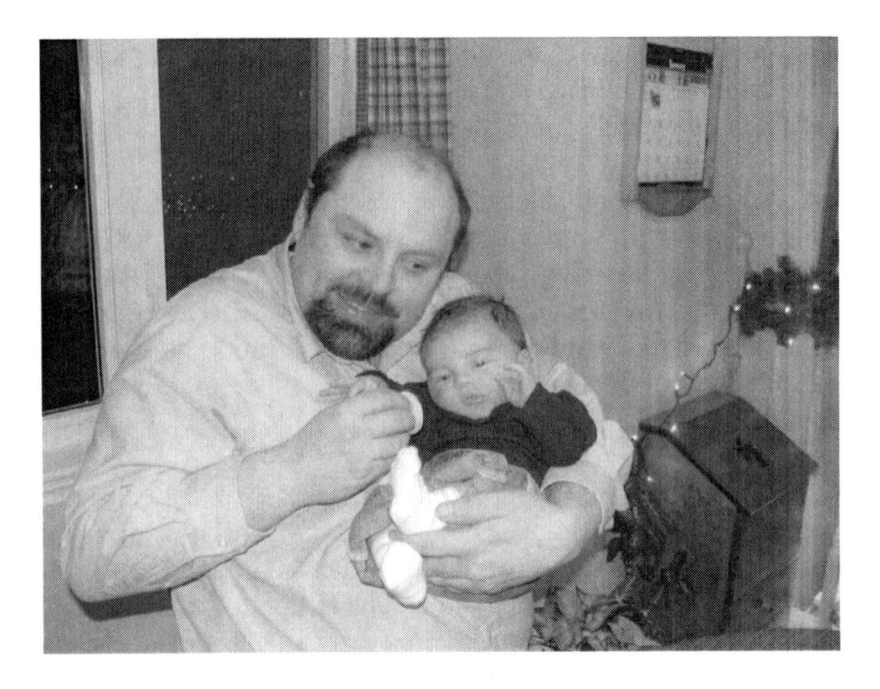

During these years in college, I made no attempt to manage or lose weight. Despite the fact that it was ruining my self-esteem and my social life (I was having an awful time getting dates) I still had the fatalistic approach; I didn't think I could lose it. I was, however, enjoying my school work and doing well. I am a problem-solver, and the classes and computer science subjects were all about solving problems. And talking or problems, I'm sure my parents saw me as one, a big one.

My parents differed in their approach to me. My mom was always supportive and proud of my accomplishments. Dad, on the other hand, wanted me to play in the National Hockey League. When it was apparent fairly on in my life that I was not going to feature in the NHL, he lost interest in me and focused almost exclusively on my younger brother.

While I was in college and still living at home, my parents divorced. My dad moved out of the family home. Mom was devastated; I wasn't. Given my age at the time, it didn't impact me the way that it would have done if it had happened earlier in my life. I was getting on with my life. I was even dating some, although there were no long-term relationships. At this point, I weighed at least 250.

One thing that didn't feature in my life at college was alcohol. Both my grandfathers had struggled with alcohol problems, and both my brother and I had witnessed first-hand the impact of alcohol. We were scared off. This, of course, made me a very valuable social asset in college life -- the designated driver! There were more than a few times when I had the unpleasant task of cleaning up my car.

Apart from being a willing and competent designated driver, I did well in my courses. This was going to stand me in good stead when I finally graduated and was ready to enter the workforce. When I was ready, the economy was in the midst of a tech boom, and I had several companies eagerly competing for my services.

I decided to accept a great job within the Canadian government. This required a move to Ottawa. For the first time, I was out of the house and, finally, independent.

Ottawa is a great city, and my job paid well. I also now had total control over my eating. I was eating out five nights a week and ordering in the other two. I was eating a lot of pizza, often overeating to the point of extreme discomfort.

I knew my weight was increasing, but my view was that I can't lose it so I might as well keep going. Again, I could find no evidence that it was possible to lose weight and keep it off, especially as I had now ballooned to over 300. The only successful example I could find was Jared from Subway, and I knew he was being aided and trained by Michael Phelps. But ordinary people can't lose this much weight and keep it off. There's no point trying.

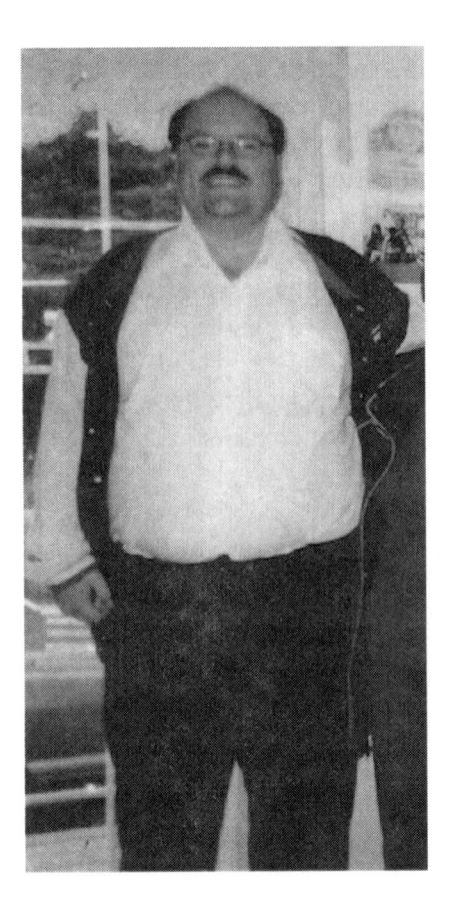

That was my attitude for the next fifteen years. I have to admit I did buy a treadmill once and used it twice, but aside from that, it was business as usual. The impact on confidence and self-esteem were there, but the confidence that I could actually do it was completely absent. I like logic. I work logically every day, and the evidence simply wasn't there. And the constant physical and social discomfort couldn't overcome this lack of scientific evidence.

I had constant reminders that I was an outcast, an object of ridicule.

One time I was walking down Bank Street, a big thoroughfare in the heart of Ottawa, with my mother. There were some college students on a balcony overlooking the street. As I passed below them one of them shouted at me, "Hey Fatso, you're not meant to eat a whole bucket of lard." I was devastated. If I sat on a bus, which I rode regularly, many people would scowl at me or give me disgusted looks for taking up the whole seat and forcing others to stand.

It hurt. I didn't show it. I didn't vent it. I stuffed it. I bottled it up. It filled me up.

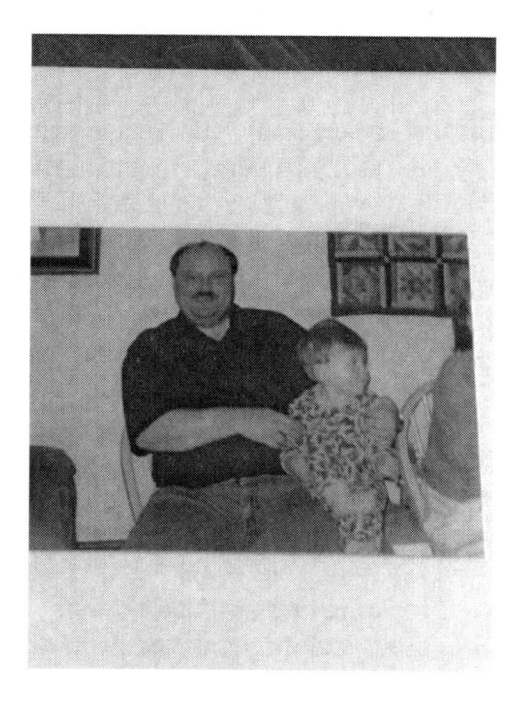

During these years, my mom was my only mentor, and she was struggling too. She didn't handle the divorce very well, and on top of that, she was also laid off from the company she had worked at for 20 years. Her eating was out of control, and her weight was going up, which was soon to have very negative consequences.

I got a promotion at work and I graduated from a programmer to being a supervisor. I became close to several of my charges. We'd often hang out together and got into the habit of playing cards at lunchtime. I also became close to one of the guys in our group. His name was Salim, and we'd occasionally hang out or go to watch boxing. Salim was into fitness, and he was often going to the gym. One week, a lot of my team were on vacation, and I had no one to hang out and play cards with.

Salim suggested that I come to the gym with him. I really didn't want to, of course. I was resigned to having a heart attack before I was fifty. He could see the same possibility, and he was more concerned about doing something about it than I was.

But, Salim was persistent and basically grabbed me by the scruff of the neck and marched me to the gym.

The first day I did a very leisurely ride on the stationary bike and was completely exhausted after twenty minutes. The next day I did the same thing, and it was a little easier. After the first week, I did feel better. I had a bit more energy. I had even lost a few pounds. So I went back the second week and lost some more weight and gained more energy. I was getting some very funny looks from the jocks at the gym, but I couldn't deny I was feeling better. Most of all, I was feeling better about myself. I was proud of my accomplishment.

After another week or two, I started to entertain the possibility that maybe I could lose some weight. Maybe not all of it, but enough to make a difference. I suffered from some serious leg ulcers as a result of poor circulation. My blood pressure was very high. My doctor recorded it at 190/130 during one visit and promptly put me on three medications. Climbing just one flight of stairs was brutal. Now, I had the glimpse of hope that maybe I could make some of that better. I might not be able to lose all the weight but maybe enough to cause a change.

After a few weeks of exercise, I could feel the difference. Now, having got some positive results, I was ready to make more of a commitment. I'd obviously need to change my eating, and that meant learning about nutrition. I had no idea what I was meant to be eating or how. Where to turn? Mom, of course.

I called her, and she told me the name of a national weight loss support group, TOPS, that she had found helpful. She had at various times been a group leader there and was very committed to the organization. I discovered that TOPS had a chapter that met weekly in a church just around the corner from where I was living.

I made a point of attending the next scheduled meeting and was given a food journal and told to plot my calorie intake. I'm a techie, not a pencil and paper guy, so started to track my intake digitally. I had no idea how much I was eating. I soon found out that I was eating about 5000 calories a day.

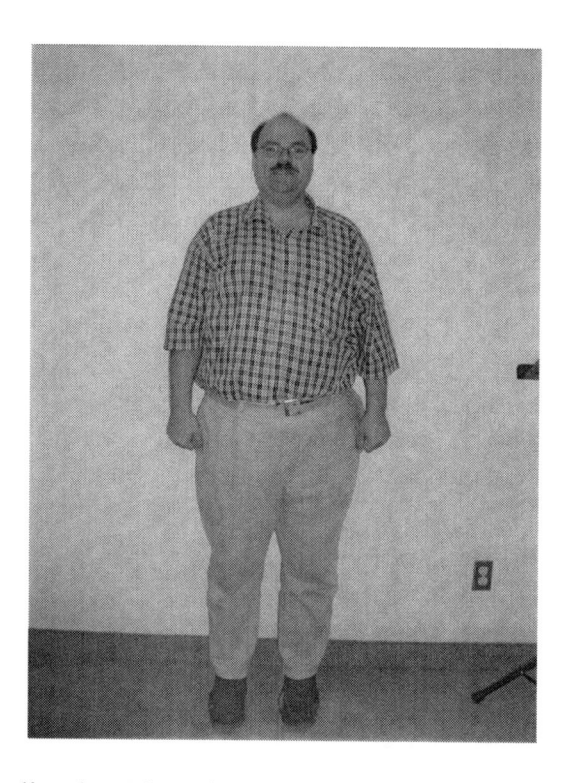

I told you earlier that I loved solving logical puzzles. I enjoy coming up with new solutions. Now, I was playing my most important game. How can I replace the foods I had been eating to save calories?

I started to replace chips and candy with popcorn while watching TV. Then I replaced French fries with steamed vegetables. I reviewed my weekly logs to seek every opportunity to make healthier choices.

I relished the challenge. How can I reduce more this week? The TOPS group was giving me great support as well as suggestions as to where I could make more nutritional economies. Finally, at age

37, I was committed to a weight-loss plan. It was the early summer of 2009.

It's a policy of my support group to get a doctor to sign off on a specific weight goal. So, after about three months, I made an appointment.

When I told him I needed him to give me a goal, he refused. He said that it would only depress me and probably demotivate me. He would prefer- as he said- to give me a small goal to reach at first. Something that was significant but manageable over a few months. He looked at my chart. I had been 350 when I last weighed in a few weeks earlier.

"Let's shoot for 315. That would be a great first step," he said.

"That doesn't work for me," I said.

The doctor looked puzzled and maybe even a bit miffed.

"What do you mean it doesn't work for you?" he said with some annoyance.

"I think I'm already there," I said.

The doc looked shocked.

"Prove it to me," he said in disbelief, as he motioned me to get on the scale.

He moved the weight back and forth to get a reading.

"You're right!" he said with a smile. 'You're already at 310!"

I had dropped 40 pounds in three months. It obviously wasn't immediately noticeable but there was no denying the progress. Honestly, it took me a while to notice the changes in me as well. Some of my co-workers could see it, and they encouraged me. It was unreal. It was the first time in my life that I was getting compliments!

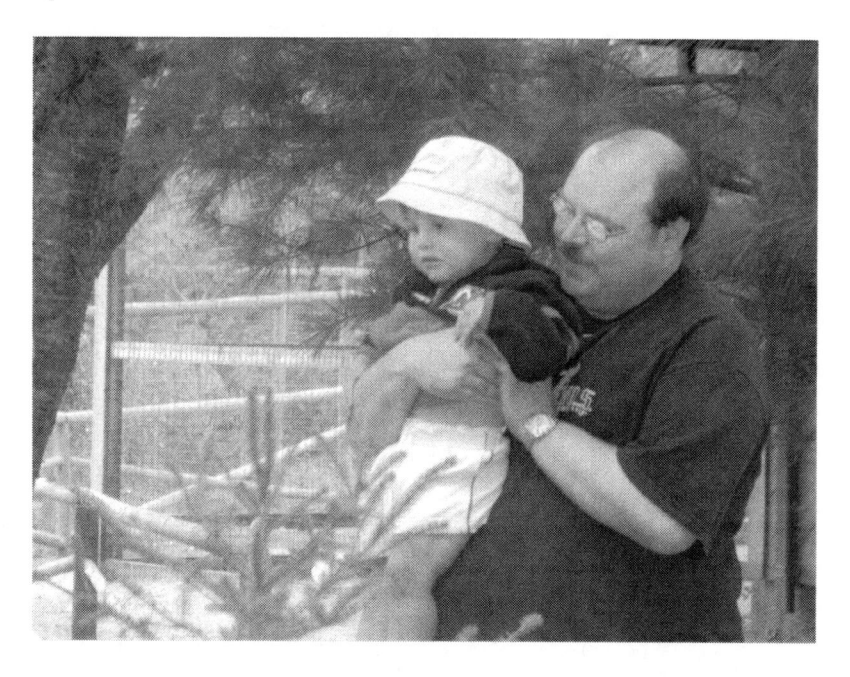

To complement my work-outs, I took up swimming. I took out a membership at a local pool. I started out very slowly doing about 20 minutes and gradually, over time, increased how long I would be in the pool. Then I increased the intensity of the swim. Of course, I needed to have data on my efforts and kept track of everything on an app called LoseIt. The app told me how many calories I should be eating and as the weight dropped off, it was telling me to eat fewer calories. I compensated by increasing my exercise output.

By this time, I was losing 4 to 5 pounds a week.

Once I was under 300 pounds I bought myself a Wii. The Wii Fit had a warning that anyone over 300 pounds shouldn't stand on the device, so I was the heaviest possible user. The Wii Fit tracked BMI and I was excited to see my Body-Mass index go down. When I first got on the scale, the Wii told me I was severely obese.

One of my proudest moments came in the spring of 2010. I weighed myself on the Wii then headed off to my TOPS meeting.

"I have something exciting to tell you all," I said. The group waited with baited breath.

"I'm FINALLY overweight!"

The Wii told me that my BMI was now below 30, the cut-off point for obesity, and I was now in the overweight category.

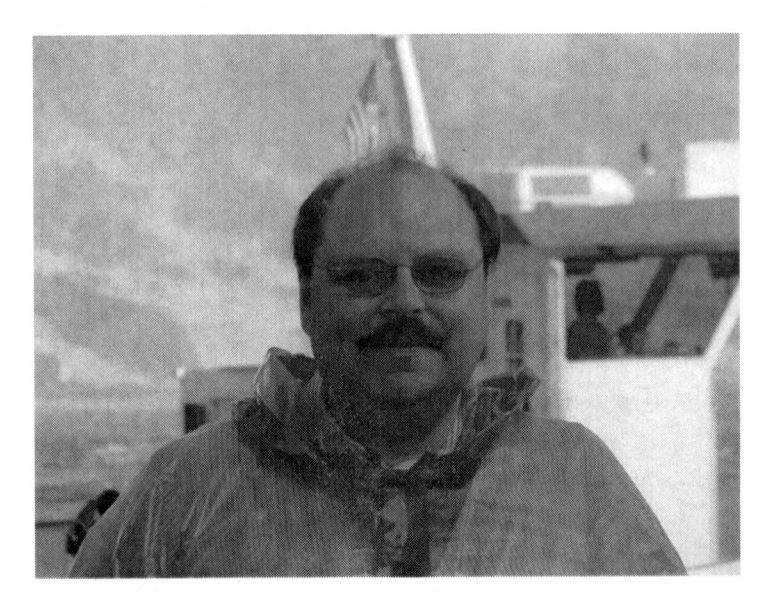

Soon after, I came into some money when a relative died and left me a modest inheritance. One thing I wanted to do is to give my mother a gift, especially since the relative was actually closer to her but hadn't let her anything.

I knew it had been my mother's dream to visit the Grand Canyon, but the cost of the trip had always been out of reach. I called my mom, and she was thrilled at the prospect. I duly made all the arrangements. We were to meet in the Toronto airport. She was flying in from Halifax, and I was coming from Ottawa.

My mother hadn't seen me in a year. I saw her as I was approaching our designated meeting point. She was looking all around for me. She didn't recognize me! It was only when I started walking towards her did she realize that it was me. I had lost over a hundred pounds. She was overwhelmed. She cried. We had a great time visiting the Grand Canyon area; especially hiking together through the various canyons.

Soon afterwards, in the spring of 2010 and about nine months into my weight loss voyage of transformation, I was visiting Halifax again. I was visiting my mother but also attending the annual meeting of TOPS.

The keynote speaker was a motivational businessman. He was talking about the importance of setting goals. His personal example was setting the goal of running a marathon. He spoke about it with such passion that I decided there and then that I was going to run a half marathon. Me, who had never run anywhere in my life. Me, who took an hour to get to first base! Yes, I decided to run more than 13 miles.

I obviously needed to build some endurance, so I signed up for a class that would gradually get me in shape by slowly increasing my distances.

The first phase was running two kilometers. I didn't find that too difficult so the next week I reported for the next phase up -- five kilometers. Again, this wasn't terribly taxing so I stepped it up the following week to the ten kilometer run. The same thing happened again, so the next week I found myself running fifteen kilometers. I was running with someone who was extolling the virtues of long-distance running.

"How long have you been running," he asked.

"This is my fourth week," I replied. The fellow was clearly shocked that I was running about 10 miles after only four weeks of running. Evidently, all that swimming I had been doing had built up my endurance. I was thrilled and also a little shocked at how well I was doing.

Less than a year after committing to run a race, and only two years after weighing 350 pounds, I ran my first half-marathon- fittingly enough- in Milwaukee, at the home of TOPS.

By then I already met my goal weight. I achieved that in August of 2010, thirteen months after starting at the gym with Salim.

I lost 180 pounds in thirteen months.

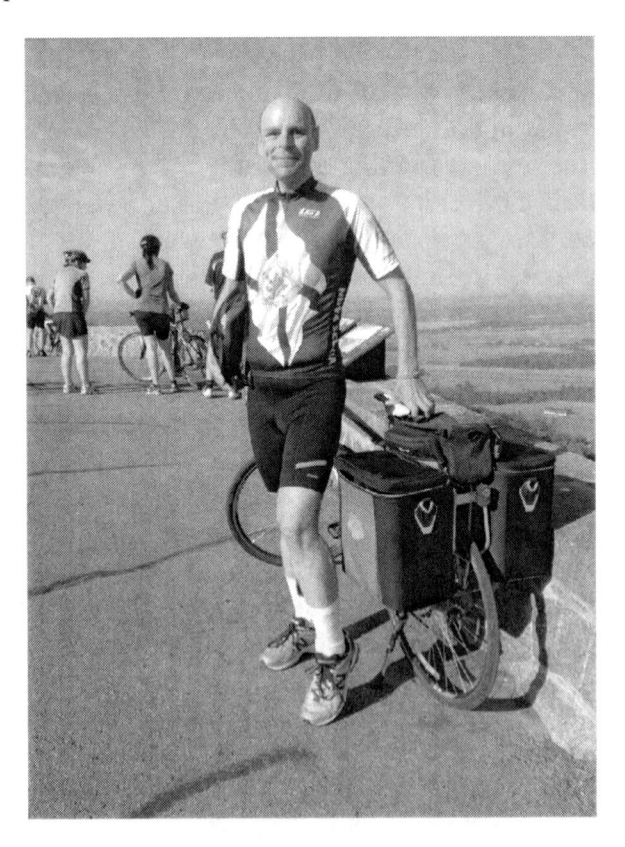

I am not sure that rate of weight loss is advisable. It certainly confused some people who knew me. The fact that I decided to shave my head at the same time added to the confusion. The simultaneous loss of hair and weight led some people to the wrong conclusion.

A neighbor who hadn't seen me put two and two together and asked me whether my cancer was in remission.

Co-workers who hadn't seen me for a year or two were also the focus of some pranks. I was sitting in one meeting and a colleague who hadn't seen me for a while was asking the others in attendance where I was. The others played along.

"I saw Don earlier, and he said he was going to be here," one of them said.

"It's unlike Don to be late," said the unsuspecting colleague.

"Perhaps you should step out to call him," another person suggested.

As she was about to step out I revealed myself!

"I'm over here," I waved.

We all had a good laugh about it. A laugh about my weight. For the right reasons.

Another time, I was getting a ride with some strangers over to a conference and one of the people said "Would you mind taking the middle seat in the back since you're the skinniest one here?" I was, like, "Now THERE is a string of words I have never heard directed my way before in my life." I almost asked her to repeat it, so I could record it on my iPhone.

There's still part of me that will always be connected to the experience of being fat.

Once I was sitting at a bar with a friend and his soccer team pals when an overweight woman came in. One of the guys said, "Humph. Look at her! Fat people really bother me.... lazy slobs." It took all my willpower not to bop him one... but I realized that I still see myself as overweight, and he was insulting me as much as her. But I later told a friend that I felt like a spy for the fat people at the thin people's meeting. "I get to hear what the thin people say when they get together, and can report back to my overweight brethren." My TOPS club connections run very deep and it isn't about being fat or skinny, it's about helping each other and respecting each other.

Crossing the finish line at that half-marathon at the home of TOPS in Milwaukee in 2011 was an emotional moment for me. It redefined who I was. I was now a runner. I was fit not fat. It felt like I had finally left that fat guy behind. This is me now. I committed myself to never being fat again.

I had so much more energy. I started to live. I was going out at nights, not stuck in front of the TV. I was dating. I was living.

In 2011, I started doing motivational speaking about my journey. I had been featured in two local newspapers, the TOPS magazine, and my workplace's newsletter; people wanted to hear my story. For my part, I wanted to give back. I knew how I suffered for so many years because I saw no example of success, had no role model, no inspiration. That was so critical for me that if I could help one person by talking about my experience, I would talk as much as I could. So, I do as many speaking engagements as I can get, which right now, is about 25 a year.

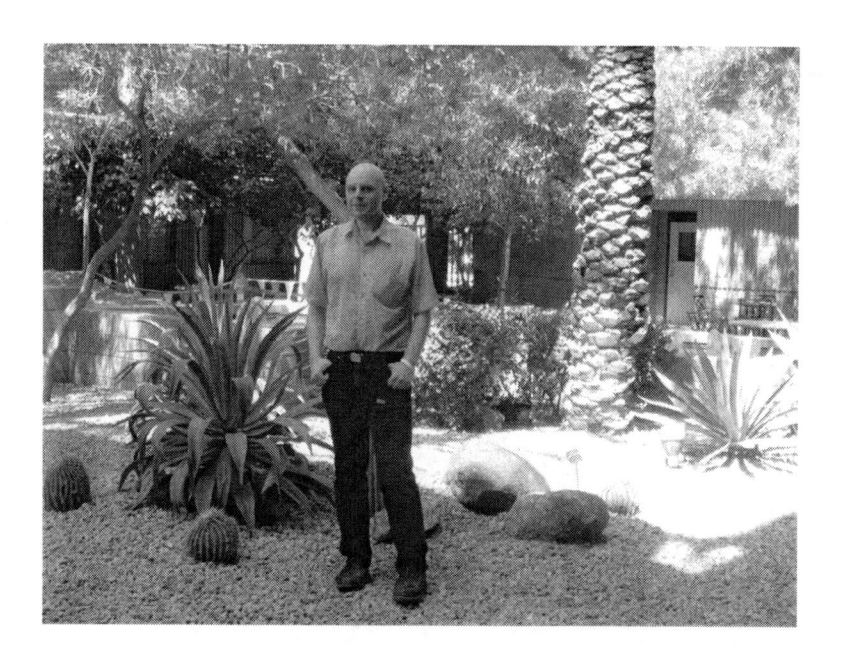

Maintenance is tough, and those speaking engagements help me as much as I hope they help others. There's nothing like public commitment for accountability. But maintenance is like a second job; you have to work really hard at it without the fun of watching the weight come off. I spend Sunday afternoons reviewing my performance in the past week, looking for ways to improve and preparing meals and meal plans. I'm aware that disaster potentially lurks around every corner.

In 2012, I struggled a lot. There were significant cutbacks that had to be made, and nobody's job was safe. In effect, we were all competing against each other -- many of us who had been friends and colleagues for years. It was a situation where if you keep your job, you feel survivor guilt, because you know that it was at the expense of a friend who has a mortgage and a family. On the other hand, losing your job would be worse. The morale at work was awful. I kept my job, but I was struggling.

Faced with this uncertainty and stress, my eating wavered, and I gained ten pounds. I was feeling like a failure until my doctor pointed out that I had gone from 350 to 180, and that was nothing to feel ashamed about. Oh, I also just ran my first marathon. That perspective helped. And so did another suggestion that he made.

He also suggested I cut out all sugar.

The first month was difficult. But once I weaned my body off sugar I have to say that total abstinence was easier than perfect moderation. I didn't realize how much sugar there was in everything that I was eating, not the obvious foods. For example, sugar was the second ingredient in the pizza sauce I was occasionally having. It was tough avoiding the cookies and cakes in the break room at work. But I knew if I didn't have the first one, I wouldn't get to ten, whereas if I did eat the first one....

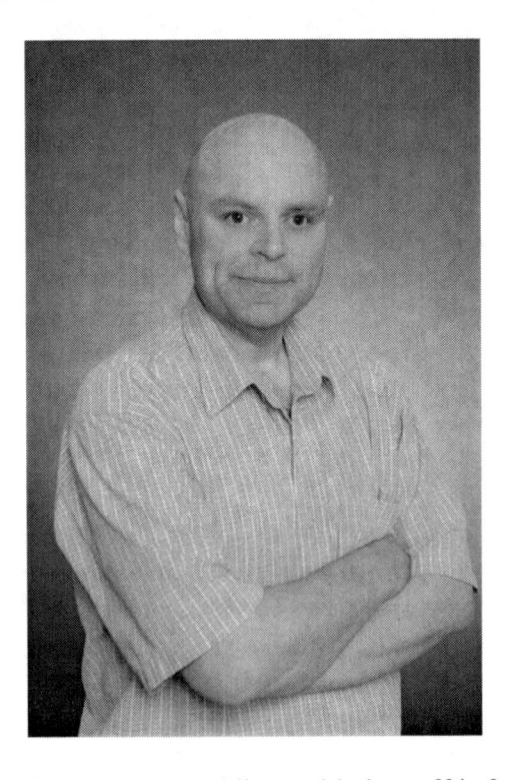

I do believe that I am a sugar addict and being off it for the past year has made maintenance so much easier. It's interesting looking back at my grandfather's difficulties with alcohol and my decision to avoid that. Alcohol is almost entirely sugar, so I suspect I might well have had a problem if I had started drinking. I could see some parallels. For example, when I used to wake in the middle of the night, I would find myself in the kitchen eating some sugary snack. So with my grandfathers' alcohol problems and my grandmother's diabetes issues, getting off sugar was definitely a good move.

When I'm giving my talks, everyone wants to know my food plan. I normally don't tell them because I think each person is an individual, and you have to work out which plan is best for you. For example, right now, I'm trying to build muscle mass, so I need protein. There's a lot of confusing and contradictory nutritional information out there. I suggest you get professional advice and customize it to your own, personal situation.

I honestly believe I lost the weight too quickly, and it wrecked my metabolism. I'd strongly encourage anyone to lose about 1-2 pounds a week not 3-4. Enjoy the journey. Actually, you are going to need to enjoy the journey because it's going to last a long time.

I met Dr. Sharma, a Canadian obesity expert, a couple of years ago. He explained that the more weight you lose, the more you are pulling away from your metabolic set-point. He conceptualized that struggle as pulling on an elastic band. The further you are from your set-point, the more drive there is to pull you back towards that set-point. Maintenance, therefore, requires holding on tight to the end of the band to prevent being catapulted back towards your set-point.

I asked Dr. Sharma whether I would always have to struggle against that set point forever

"No, not forever," he said, "Only until you die. Which will likely be a long time away should you keep the weight off."

There's one other thing about my diet you do need to know.

Crazy binges with cheeseburgers in my teen years notwithstanding, I have been a vegetarian since my late teens. You don't have to be on high fat diet to gain weight. There is such a thing as an unhealthy vegetarian diet. I was eating way too many carbs. When people express surprise that I was a 350-pound vegetarian, I tell them I've changed my diet from pizza, pasta and pie to beans, broccoli and bananas. I have added a lot more protein and cut out the high glycemic carbs. It has worked for me.

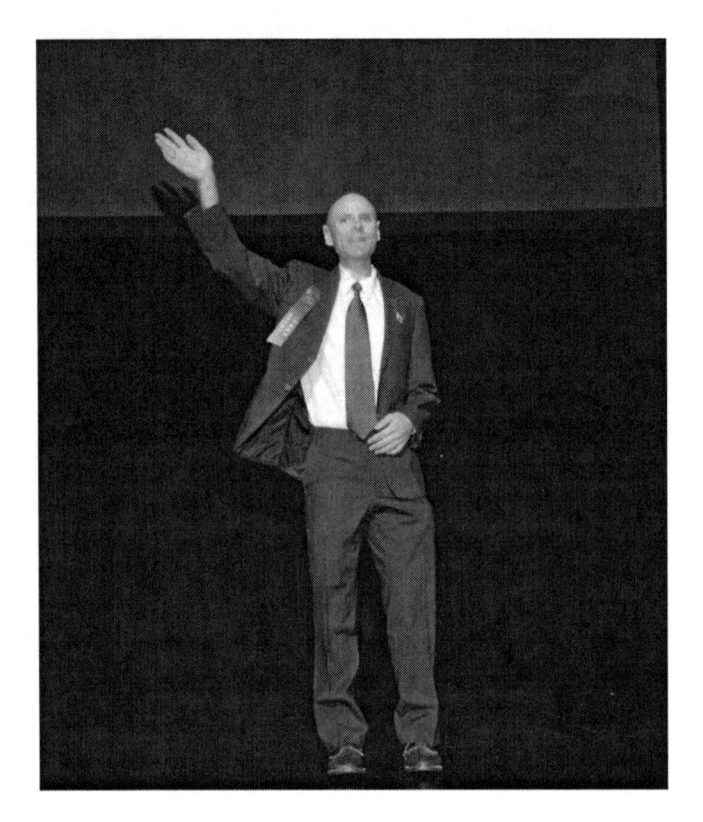

I believe that mentors and inspiration are critical for success. I can't give enough thanks to my fiend Salim, who forced me to the gym five years ago and changed my life. At his retirement party, I was able to honor and acknowledge Salim for his role in turning my life around. My life has changed, and I have grown so much because of him. I've climbed one of the Rocky Mountains, and I ran my first marathon last year, in my hometown of Halifax. And Salim is not just responsible for the change in my weight and fitness but also my psyche. For example, I now have self-confidence. I can speak in public, something I would have been horrified to do a few years ago. I told Salim at that retirement party, "I had no idea that as my body would shrink, that I would grow so much bigger as a person. And that I owe him not just for likely adding years to my life, but making the time between now and when I pass to be BETTER years."

That's why I want to give back and help others on their way just as Salim helped me. It's really important to me to help others. Only last week I just got chills down my spine when a woman came up to me and said she had heard me speak six months ago, and I had inspired her to start running.

"I feel so much better, and I'm down two dress sizes!" she said.

I always said that if I could inspire just ONE person the way that Salim motivated me, then my efforts would be worth it. But I always secretly hoped that one person would be my mother. She has always been the most supportive and loving influence in my life. A couple of years ago, her type II diabetes significantly worsened. She had to check her blood sugar levels constantly. I was really concerned about her. I have given her the tools and the encouragement, but she has been putting in the effort to improve her health, and at the time of writing; she is now down sixty pounds. And her diabetes has virtually disappeared, and her doctor has given her the go-ahead to stop checking her blood sugar.

Since I had gone from being 350 pounds to about 175, the running joke at work was that "I was half the man I used to be." I would laugh at the joke, but I got to that it was nowhere near the truth. Looking back on my life, I am twice the man who used to spend his evenings and weekends watching TV and stuffing his face.

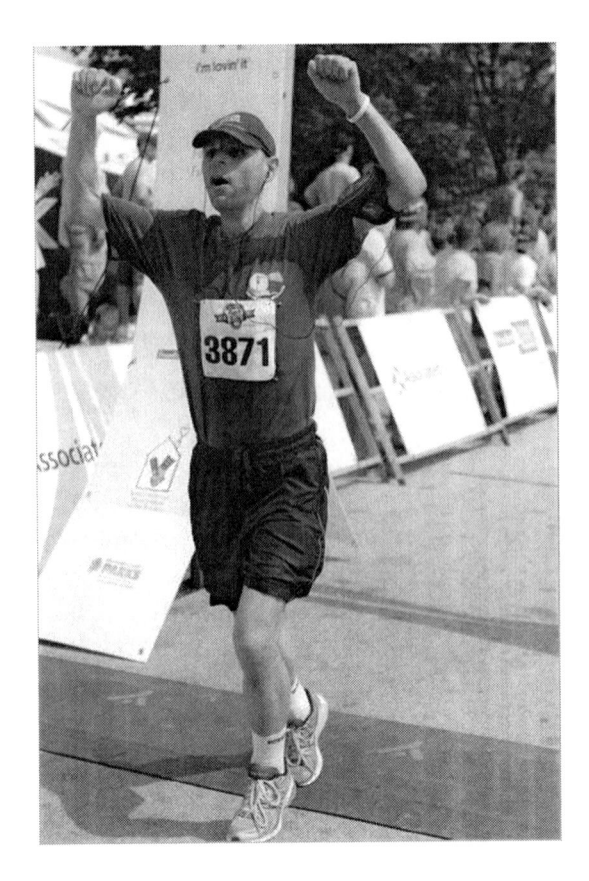

I am not half the man I used to be, only half the MASS I used to be. So that is what I have named my Facebook page and my blog (halfthemassIusedtobe.wordpress.com).

Toye Seales

Eating for Two

While I was growing up, I was very active. I always had a lot of drive, and I loved to dance and play. Despite the fact that some of my family were overweight, dieting was never on my radar screen. Blessed with a great metabolism and a lot of energy, I ate what I wanted, and I was never overweight. On the contrary, at a little more than 5'6" and consistently weighing in at around 120, I was in great shape. I was in such great shape that I even did some modeling. I got used to being in front of a camera, and I have to admit; I liked being the center of attention. At this time in my life, my early twenties, I loved dressing up in colorful clothing and high heels that drew plenty of looks. It was fun and the notion of being overweight or even eating healthily was not part of my consciousness at all.

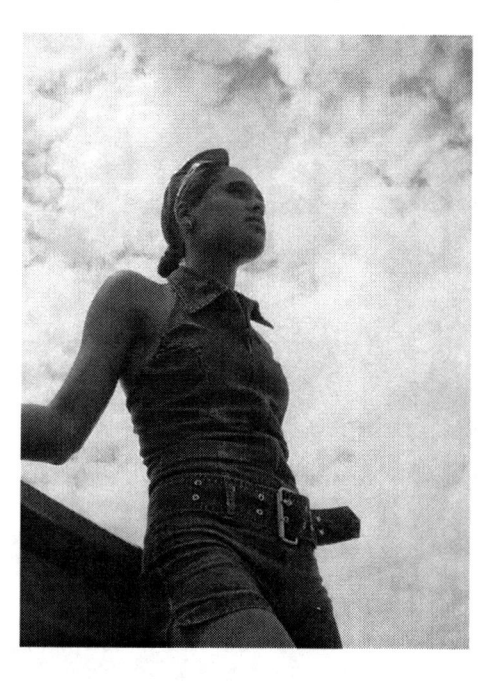

When I was twenty-eight and still enjoying life as a svelte young adult that still loved to dance and have plenty of energy, I became pregnant. I was so excited! There didn't seem any reason to change my behavior much. I was in great shape. In fact, during the first six months of my pregnancy, I hardly gained any weight, and my pregnancy didn't really show until at least twenty weeks. In the last trimester, the excess weight suddenly started to appear. My doctor told me that in the last trimester a gain of about one pound a week was desirable but there were weeks when I was gaining seven pounds. By the time I delivered Taniqa (the name means 'Beauty') I had actually gained sixty pounds, almost all in the last three months.

I wasn't too worried. I knew this weight was a result of my pregnancy, and that I could now set about losing it. My physician, however, had other ideas. He said that while I was breastfeeding Taniqa, I shouldn't go on a diet. I could be active and even exercise but reducing my calorie intake while breastfeeding wasn't a good idea, he advised. I wasn't fazed. I continued to eat a lot of junk food, eat out a lot and drink four liters of Pepsi a day.

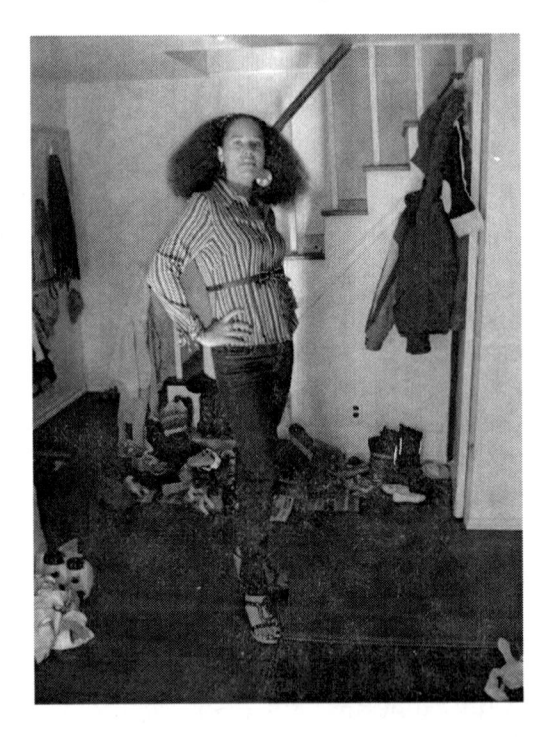

I breastfed Taniqa for a year. During that time, I gained another fifteen pounds but again in my mind; I wasn't really fat -- just carrying the after-effects of being pregnant. As I finished breastfeeding Taniqa, I headed back to the doctor to get some advice on how to lose the more than seventy pounds I had gained. That's when I discovered I was pregnant again!

My second pregnancy was very similar to my first. I didn't gain much early on, but the weight piled on in the third trimester. I didn't gain as much as the first pregnancy, about forty as opposed to the sixty pounds, but it was now added to the seventy, or so, that was left over from the first pregnancy.

Tashi (the name means 'Pride') was also a natural birth and normal delivery. However, with both Taniqa and Tashi, I did have some gestational diabetes.

Again, my physician advised that I should not try to reduce my calorie intake or go on a diet while I was breastfeeding Tashi. I was unfazed again. In a funny sort of way, I didn't see the extra weight as my weight. But after I continued to gain a few pounds while breastfeeding Tashi, it suddenly hit me. Here I was about a hundred pounds heavier than I had ever been. I had never been overweight in my life. Moreover, now I wasn't getting any of the looks or attention that I was so used to having. In fact, I wasn't getting any attention at all!

I became pretty depressed. There seemed to be a mismatch between my inner sense of myself and how others were now reacting to me. On the inside, I was still the fun, energetic person I had always been, but people were not reacting to me that way. Needless to say, I couldn't fit into any of my clothes. Not only that, but I couldn't even find the sort of clothes I was used to wearing. They didn't come in my new, enhanced size. It got to the point where I hated to be seen. Whereas before I had been the energetic center of attention, now I couldn't even get myself out of the door. Where I used to love being in front of the camera, now I didn't want anyone to take my photo. Seriously, there are no photos of me during this time.

When I stopped breastfeeding Tashi, after about nine months, I was very ready to lose the excess weight. I discussed my weight-management plans with my doctor, and soon I had joined Curves; a local gym for women just like me who were trying to get control of their weight and their fitness.

I also decided I needed some support and advice, so I joined my local TOPS (Take Off Pounds Sensibly) chapter. I got some great information and encouragement from the group and within a few weeks, I had dropped fifteen pounds and weighed in just under 200. I was on my way. Then something happened to stop me in my tracks.

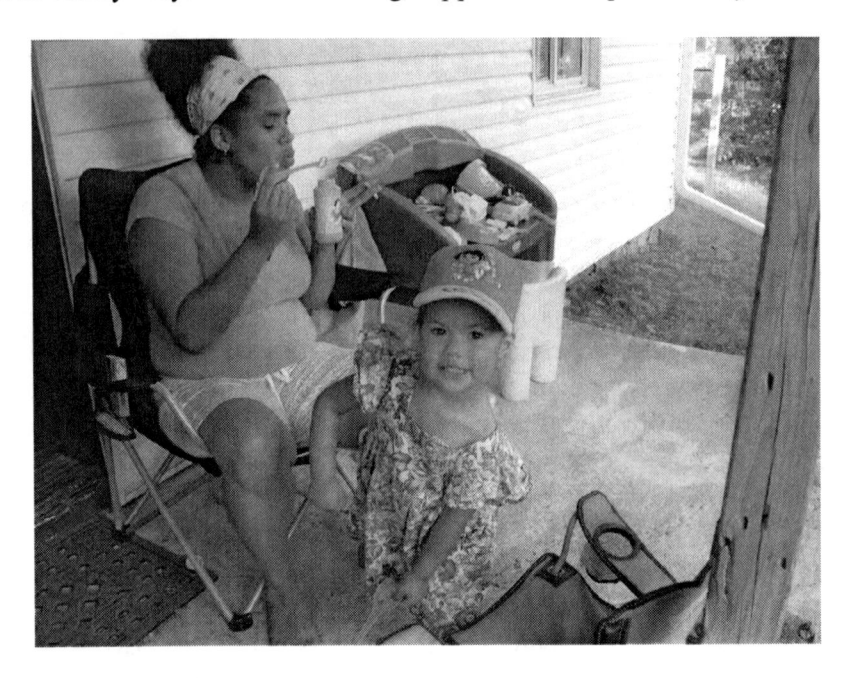

I became pregnant again. Oh no!

My pregnancy carrying Talyn (the name means 'Courage') was similar to the first two, although I was much more wary the third time around. I tried to keep up some sort of exercise, and I didn't justify that I was eating for two. I discovered that the extra nutritional demands during pregnancy amounted to about two hundred additional calories a day, not the hundreds or even thousands extra that I, and many other pregnant women, rationalize away. So, I was much more aware of my eating and made healthier substitutions wherever possible. I don't think the fact that Talyn was a boy made any difference; it was that I was just more aware. For example, I ate Fiber One chocolate bars rather than Snickers. As a result, I only gained about thirty pounds during the pregnancy.

When it was time to stop breastfeeding Talyn, I headed straight to the doctor once more and recommitted to my program. I rejoined TOPS and Curves.

Deprivation does not work for me; substitution does. I continued to look for better alternatives. One of the biggest that I was finally able to make was the switch to *diet* Pepsi.

I don't like restricting my calorie intake, and because I have a naturally high metabolism, I don't need a calorie-restricted diet. For example, 1200 calories a day wouldn't work for me, and I don't need to be that restrictive to lose weight. I was very mindful of what I was eating and making much better choices, but I didn't see this as restriction.

I really enjoyed working out. The fact that Curves wasn't competitive, helped. It wasn't home to hard-body trainers or professional fitness fanatics, just regular women trying to get in better shape. I typically was going three times a week, and I found my time there really valuable as I came to see it as time for myself, for me to focus on me.

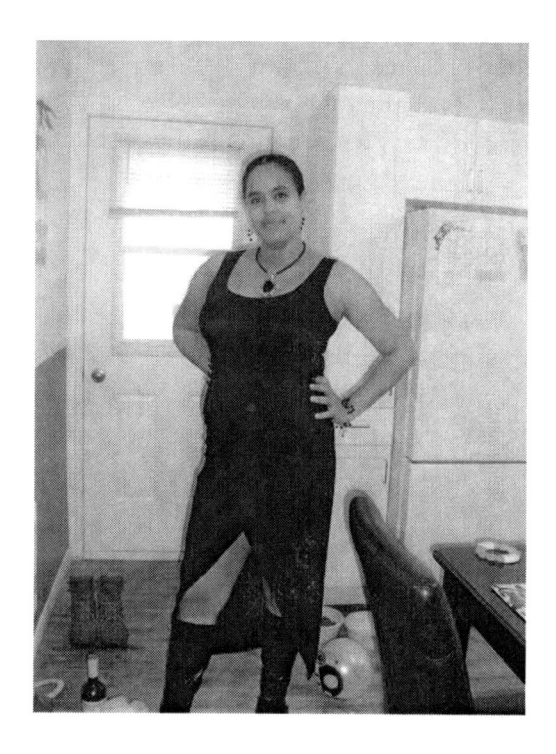

TOPS was also a great time to focus on what I needed, and I learned a lot. I saw older women who had struggled for a lifetime with their weight, and they inspired me to break the cycle now, while I was still young. The women were incredibly supportive, and they also had great information and recipes. Weighing in every week at the TOPS meeting also gave me some much-needed accountability. I also saw the struggles of many of the members and realized that because of my age and my generally good health, I was in a lot better position to tackle the weight issue than many of them. I realized that I needed to get control of my weight now, rather than delay until I might not have the energy or general health to be successful. I observed many members were struggling with years of bad habits that were proving very difficult to reverse.

I was getting support and motivation from home, too. My husband was incredibly supportive through these pregnancies and the ordeal with my escalating weight. He always told me that he loved me regardless of my weight. He is in good shape so it must have been hard for him to see his previously slim, model wife, balloon up to over two hundred pounds. I'm not sure he fully understood the impact the weight had on my psyche. He saw me as the same woman, but inside, I didn't feel like the same woman.

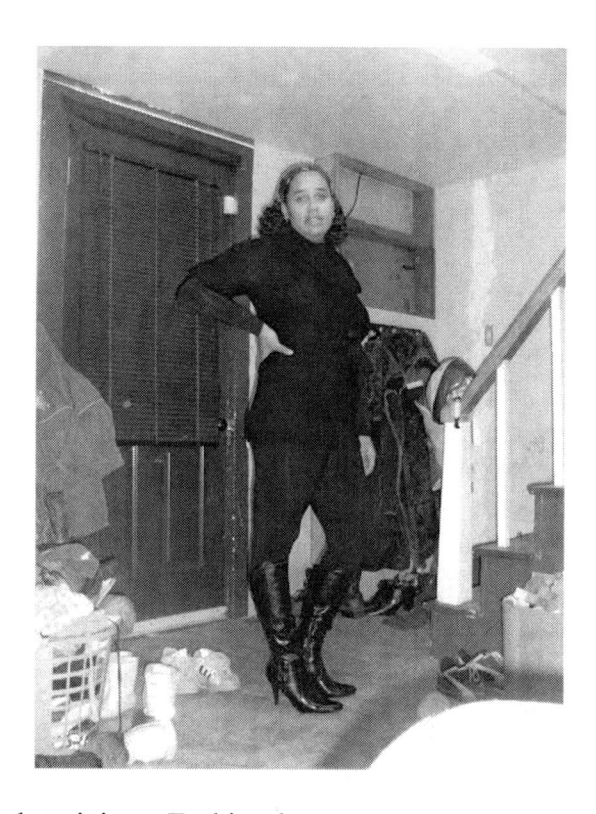

To add insult to injury, Tashi- who was now two- was providing her own opinions about her mother's size. One time she said, "Wow! Mommy your belly is all big and jiggly!"

If that wasn't motivation enough, Taniqa also told me that some of the food I was eating wasn't healthy, at least according to what she had learned in pre-school.

I continued to make healthier substitutions. For example, I would allow myself to bake my own oven fries rather than buy them from a fast-food place. Gradually, with better nutrition, working out regularly, support from TOPS and my family, the weight started to come off.

After the loss of the first ten pounds I got a refrigerator magnet to remind me of my accomplishment. After the loss of the next ten pounds, I felt some of my old energy return. I actually said to my husband, "I feel as if a little piece of Toye has come back."

When I lost some more weight, I wanted to be seen again. Inspired, I upped my attendance at Curves to five times a week and really focused on my efforts. It took me a few months, but I soon reached my goal weight, having lost more than sixty pounds.

Initially, I had visions of getting down to my modeling weight and looking like I was twenty again. I tried to get into one of my dresses from my early twenties, and it was definitely a challenge. It helped me realize that I wasn't twenty any more. I am in my mid-thirties, and I have three children. For my height, a weight of 150 gave me a Body Mass Index that was in the normal-weight range. At 150, I can wear beautiful clothes, and I can get back into those heels! I can take full pride in my appearance as I used to do. I am no longer hiding.

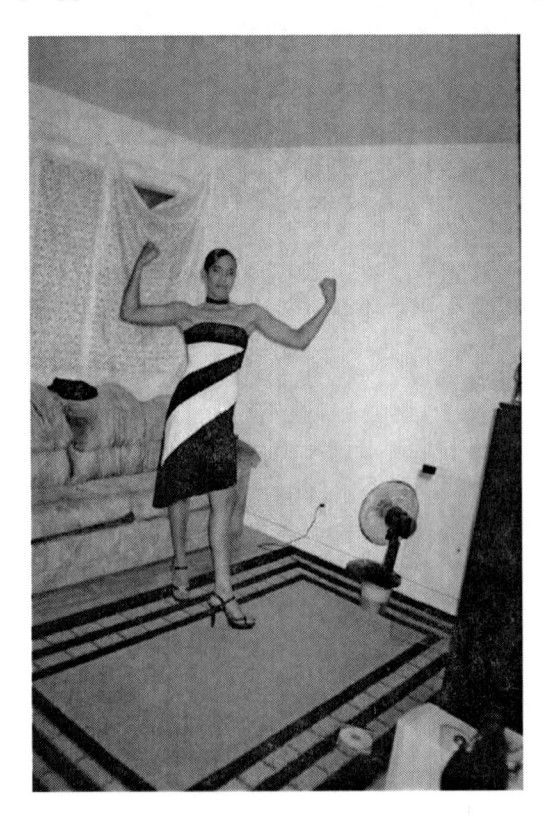

As the old Toye returned I got a little cocky. I stopped paying attention, and I paid the price. I quickly regained ten pounds. That was a very helpful warning. I have to continue to pay attention to what I eat, and I have to commit to taking care of myself through exercise. I soon got back on track and lost the ten pounds I had carelessly gained.

At TOPS, I became a chapter leader, which helped me in two ways. It enabled me to give back to the organization, and it also helped my focus on my efforts. In 2013, I was the TOPS Queen for the province of Quebec. This led to my appearance at the 2014 annual TOPS convention in Milwaukee where I was recognized as the weight loss leader in my province. I had a great time and even got the opportunity to lead thousands of the attendees in a Zumba class.

On reflection, my journey is about several important issues. One is self-deception. It is so easy to fool yourself into rationalizing away your weight problem. In my case, it didn't help that I had physicians telling me that I shouldn't diet but, of course, they were telling me to eat sensibly and exercise. Pregnancy provides a great excuse for eating whatever you want but let me tell you categorically "eating for two" isn't necessary and sooner or later, you have to face the consequences.

I am also a great believer in finding your own way and using the tools and techniques that work for you. There is no magic bullet, and one size doesn't fit everybody. For me, healthy substitutions worked really well, along with regular exercise. To be effective, I had to pay attention to my behavior and especially my eating, but I could eat more healthily without restricting. Because I took this approach, I never really felt that I was on a diet, but that I really was making a lifestyle change.

Support was a critical element in my change, and I am sure everyone needs it when they are trying to change any behavior. The support I got helped me stay accountable, realize in some ways how lucky I was, and also gave me great information and advice.

During my worst times, life became pretty dark, and I lost myself. I have learned that you cannot allow yourself to get lost. You must pay attention to your health and self because no one else will. It's a message I will definitely share with my three beautiful children.

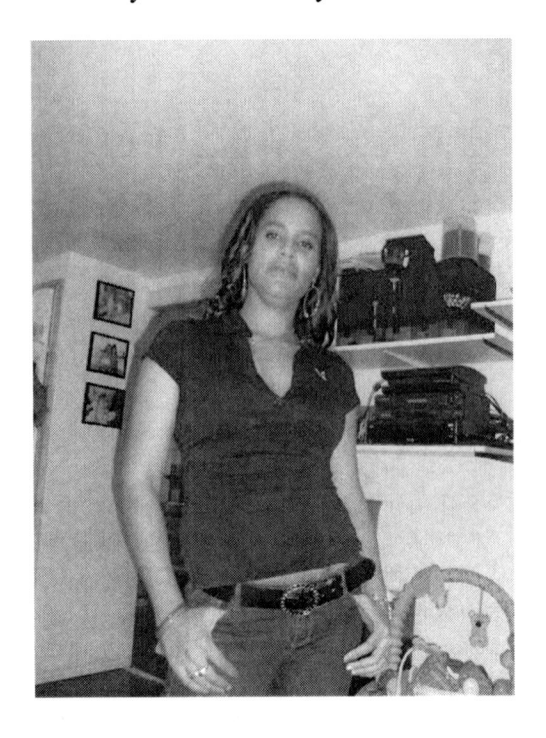

Andrea Martinez

From the Negative to the Positive

I grew up in Miami, the child of immigrants from Cuba. My parents came to the United States when they were pre-teens, but they carried with them the legacy of their upbringing. That legacy was simply the fact, that food was a precious commodity which needed to be eaten when available, and that a few extra pounds were a sign of status...and survival. As a result, food was valued obsessively in my house. There simply was a primitive need to eat first and do other things later. Calories were not just a priority; they were *the* priority.

I remember many times as a child being forced to eat when I was no longer hungry. But, I would go along with it, because I wasn't allowed to do anything else until I had eaten everything on my plate. It may not be a surprise for you to learn that my family was borderline obese. And I was huge. I was always the biggest in my class -- and probably the most self-conscious.

I weighed over 100 pounds before I even got to elementary school -- the largest kid in the class. I became very nice to others; it was the only thing I thought I had going for me. I saw myself as ugly, so being friendly and helpful was the only thing I could offer. I have that problem even to this day. People still take advantage of me because I'm too nice. But, my helpfulness softened the rejection and the bullying. I did have friends, but they'd make fun of me, too. I'd blow it off and laugh with them. In a state of denial, I thought I was just chubby, but I felt a heavier burden than that.

My parents just didn't know about proper nutrition. To be fair, it was all about carbs back then, and that's about all I got. Tons of them; with some high-fat protein thrown in for good measure.

My parents also ate this diet, of course, and they became the ultimate yo-yo dieters. My mom, in particular, went on every diet imaginable. She went to Weight Watchers, obsessively. At times, I thought she looked anorexic. She once lost over 100 pounds but regained it all back and then some. My dad has always been obese, and his father is obese, too.

Not only did my parents struggle with their weight and were uneducated about proper nutrition, they didn't know how to address my problem. They simply didn't really have a proper conversation with me about it at all. They would bribe me. My mom said she would buy me new clothes if I lost weight, but then fed me the same diet! My dad really didn't talk to me about it and then one day just suddenly stopped our morning routine of going to Dunkin' Donuts. I didn't know why.

Mom went to Weight Watchers and bought their foods, but they were for her not me. I kept being fed the fundamentally wrong foods. For example, I was still being given mac and cheese but the ham had been removed. They just didn't know.

There was a time when my mother's mom was looking after me, and things weren't any better. In fact, she would take me to McDonald's every day, after school. I think that's when I reached rock bottom, physically and emotionally.

I was getting contradictory messages. For example, my grandmother -- the one taking me to McDonalds -- would scream at me "You're overweight!" She would also scream at her daughter- my mom, "She's too big!"

Everyone seemed to be making fun of me, and my self-esteem was non-existent. A friend's mother brought it up to my parents, but it didn't make any difference. They were having their own struggles. And, besides, I think they had a fatalistic view of my fat. It was all in the genes; they thought. My mom didn't take me to Weight Watchers, but she did take me to a gymnastic class for overweight kids. I loved that!

The only family time we had was either on vacation or going to a restaurant. My brother is five years younger, and even he started to gain weight in middle school. He has gone back to bad habits now, as he is busy and has a demanding job. He eats out for almost every meal!

In elementary school, I was a mess; an extra-large mess. I never had any nice clothes, and actually nothing really fit me. I had nothing fashionable. I almost always wore stretch pants and a big shirt as a cover-up.

I didn't do very well in school, and instead, focused on boosting my self-esteem by making friends, trying to be accepted-- even popular. Phys. Ed. was a big problem for me, too. I was always the last one running a lap. Miraculously, I was always absent on the day we had to climb rope, for some strange reason, -- actually a miracle. I was always last running the mile. Everyone was running it in about 8 minutes, and I was four minutes behind everyone else. I had to walk some of it. Everyone made fun of me as I crossed the finish line.

In middle school, things changed for the better. First, my standard outfit, long shorts covered up with a baggy shirt, were actually in fashion at the time, so I didn't look quite so out of place. And there were now some kids who were almost as big as I was, which helped to deflect the attention and make me feel not so much of a freak.

In middle school people seemed to change, too. They became more social and with my caring, helpful nature, I got to be included. The talk was about what was cool -- fashion, clothes, trends -- and I could participate. In fact, some kids who had been enemies in elementary school became my friends -- to a degree. I was, for example, never invited to the beach with the really cool kids. Moreover, my parents' over- protectiveness didn't help. They wouldn't let me socialize after school hours, which certainly stunted my social development. One time, I do remember having a pool party at my home, but that was the big adventure (I am sure I wore a big shirt over my bathing suit.) Moreover, the Cuban culture dictated that girls should be at home after school, not running around unsupervised with other kids. Nonetheless, despite these restrictions

I did, much to my surprise, attract the interest of a couple of boys. It never amounted to anything, but it felt good to know that there were some boys who found this fat girl attractive.

In my freshman high school year, I sank into a big depression. There were a lot of negative things happening, and with the advance in social graces that comes at that age, people were one again making fun of me and eating away at my fragile self-esteem. But, I continued to try to be popular and still, of course, had an interest in the boys. By the beginning of my sophomore year, I was close to 200 (I'm 5'6" tall). But, I was doing well at school -- somehow. I actually made the honor roll -- one roll I was proud of.

Then something miraculous happened. I started dating a boy on the football team. It was towards the end of ninth grade, and I was huge. I started to confide in him about my fears and my feelings, and how horrible I felt most of the time. He had a treadmill in his home, and he started to teach me about physical fitness.

As well as the cardio on the treadmill, my boyfriend taught me about weights. I had never, ever considered lifting weights -- I assumed only boys did that. But by the tenth grade, he was pushing me more and more. We were doing weights, running and generally doing a lot together.

By the eleventh grade, I was down to 120 pounds!! Yes, on my boyfriend's regime and what he told me about simple nutrition principles -- I was slowly learning about salads and soups and generally lighter fare -- I lost more than 60 pounds. I even became a cheerleader!

By this time, I had eliminated junk food, in fact, all fast food. I was making my own meals consisting mostly of fruit and veggies. I was hardly ever eating out. I became like my mom, obsessive, especially about the gym. I was religiously going twice a day.

Of course, I liked the fact that the weight was coming off but I was also a little conflicted. While I liked it on one hand, I fell back into cultural thinking, on the other. I was working so hard to lose it and yet telling myself, "you're too skinny."

I was an honor roll student in the tenth and eleventh grades but in the twelfth grade, I left the school structure and was in a work experience program. My first assignment was as a file clerk at an ob/gyn office at a hospital.

I lost my focus, structure and discipline. I was very stressed and it didn't help when I found out that people in the health professions aren't the best role models. They smoke, drink coffee as if its water, and even the food in the hospital cafeteria isn't healthy.

To make matters worse, things at home were very stressful. My family life wasn't very stable and I was actually shuttling between my grandmother's home and my mother's house a lot of the time. It was very stressful, and to cope; I turned to pot. Let me tell you that 'the munchies' are real. I started to eat donuts again and before long was completely off track and back to my old eating habits.

My early adulthood is a blur, a drug-induced dive into depression and desolation. I moved out on my own, and it was a huge struggle. I moved to Orlando and struggled to find work.

I went downhill fast. I hardly had any money. I was bouncing around between different full-time and part-time jobs, trying to figure out what to do. I worked as an independent contractor for Bell South, a photographer in a studio, I even had a job in property management.

I was completely lost, isolated and out-of-control. My weight ballooned. It seemed like I blew up -- literally and metaphorically -- overnight. But by now, my weight wasn't my most pressing problem. Yes, I was now 235, but I was also getting to be seriously dysfunctional. I started to have flashbacks and was referred to a psychiatrist and a psychologist. I was admitted to the hospital. While there, I was put on anti-depressants, which lifted my spirits, but -- I didn't realize at the time -- would only keep me locked into my obesity.

I moved in with my brother in Orlando and went to school at Valencia Community College. My brother was a college student, too, and he was partying it up. I, however, remained isolated in my room with my dog. Eva, my Chihuahua, was my only friend. No one would even look at me. It was terrible. I was taking my meds but also smoking pot, which limited the effectiveness of both. I couldn't get high no matter how hard I tried -- and I tried pretty hard. I didn't understand what really happens when the body is dependent on chemicals.

I'd take my frustrations out with food, of course. This miserable situation lasted for about three years. I started to regain some semblance of control and started going to the gym. However, the drugs were limiting my heart rate, and I could never get a good cardio workout. After three miserable years, much to the surprise of my family, I graduated with an Associate's degree in arts and general studies.

In Orlando, I had tried the South Beach Diet, but it didn't work for me. But now I decided it was time to return to the South Beach area itself to try to get my life back on track. I moved back to Miami.

I did actually live in South Beach on my own. It was a difficult adjustment. I did have a friend, just one, but it was a start. I decided to go back to a four-year college to finish my degree. Initially, I signed on at Berry but soon transferred to Florida International University (FIU), where I was studying photography and art history. I've always been a late bloomer, and here I was definitely one of the older students.

The structure of school forced me to get out and be social, if not sociable. I was also enjoying the artistic life, and I started to take better care of myself. I had been trying to wean of my meds for a while, but it was a long and unsuccessful process. But now I was back in Miami; I found a different doctor, and he helped me eventually got off all my medications. There are some anti-depressant and other medications, particularly older ones, that make it very difficult to lose weight, if not create weight gain outright. For whatever reason, my body wasn't just functioning right. I didn't have a menstrual period for years.

I was so happy to be off my anti-depressants! Freed from the effects of the medications, I started to eat much more sensibly and work out. The weight started to come off.

At FIU, I was still smoking pot. It helped with my creativity and my social anxiety. Using pot, seemed to improve my social life. I had to research and be involved in group projects, or go on field trips, discussions, so I was forced to participate more. The art program is very interactive, so I had to socialize. Not that socializing was easy. My mentors and fellow students were critical of me. It hurt but also helped. They told me, for example, that if you're obese it's harder to get a job. This interaction helped.

Another thing that motivated me was something I've heard many people say. However, my experience came as part of my studies. In my first year at FIU, I was doing a photography course. One project involved taking a photograph of myself. That negative was really a positive. That's when I saw myself as I really was. Up to that point, I didn't see the reality of it, and you don't until you look in the mirror. I was wearing dresses and tank tops and when I look back now, I wonder what I was thinking. I was so overweight, even though by this time I had already started losing and was down about sixty pounds from my heaviest.

I was going to the gym at FIU and eating sensibly. I was off my meds and my mood was good. I was still slightly overwhelmed and lonely, but I was in control. I had to commute; I had to go print in the darkroom at night, and was staying late hours, often eating from the vending machine, but I still managed to keep to a low calorie plan of sorts. At this time, I was drinking only water. I'm not sure where I heard it -- it could have been on Oprah (I'm a big fan) -- "it's much better to eat your calories rather than drink them." So I wasn't drinking any sodas or juices. Many people don't realize how many calories they drink. Now, I don't ever drink soda. I carry water around with me all the time.

The other critical thing that I did was educate myself. I took lifestyle modification courses at FIU. They taught me how to strike the right balance between nutrition and exercise. I took a nutrition course and started to hang out with budding nutritionists and dietitians. I saw first-hand how serious they were about everything they put in their bodies. They taught me a lot.

I learned many things from them. Cheap food is not good for you. Eat every two hours. No eating past a certain time at night. First thing in the morning, drink two cups of water before you do anything else. Eat a Greek yogurt before a meal and your stomach won't absorb as many calories.

I also enrolled in a cooking course where the classroom was divided into about ten different kitchens. Every day we had to cook a different meal with different nutrients, and I learned how cooking affects the nutrients in foods. My social interaction with these informed health-conscious people also made a huge difference.

One girl, in particular, was very health-conscious. She was really into eating organic. We became close friends, and she taught me a lot. I absorb from others. Being older than the other students, I had a naturally slower metabolism, too, and this knowledge helped me adjust my diet even more.

I lost at a steady pace at FIU. Trying to lose slowly and surely about one pound a week, I have lost over 100 pounds. I graduated with my degree in 2013. Photography is my passion.

My weight and my health are an ongoing battle. I realize how critical my environment is. I don't like to be around people that aren't healthy; they have a very negative effect on me. I have a friend now that I'm about to cut loose because all he does is eat at Burger King, and it is driving me insane!

I did a boot camp once, but I didn't like it. I prefer my own cardio work-out and weights. I lift free weights at my house.

My family is not supportive at all. I sense a lot of jealousy from both my mother and my father. My father is envious of healthy, fit bodies -- he can't get it overnight. He would need to work at it. My mother is once again on another fad diet, and is currently taking three milk shakes a day. It's a yo-yo diet.

Be patient on your weight loss journey. Don't go for yo-yo dieting. Educate yourself. It's a science: energy in- energy out. I see the weight camp, big weight loss shows -- they are too extreme. If you're 300 pounds, there are a lot of exercises that are too difficult or too uncomfortable. Don't do it. Just go for what you can do.

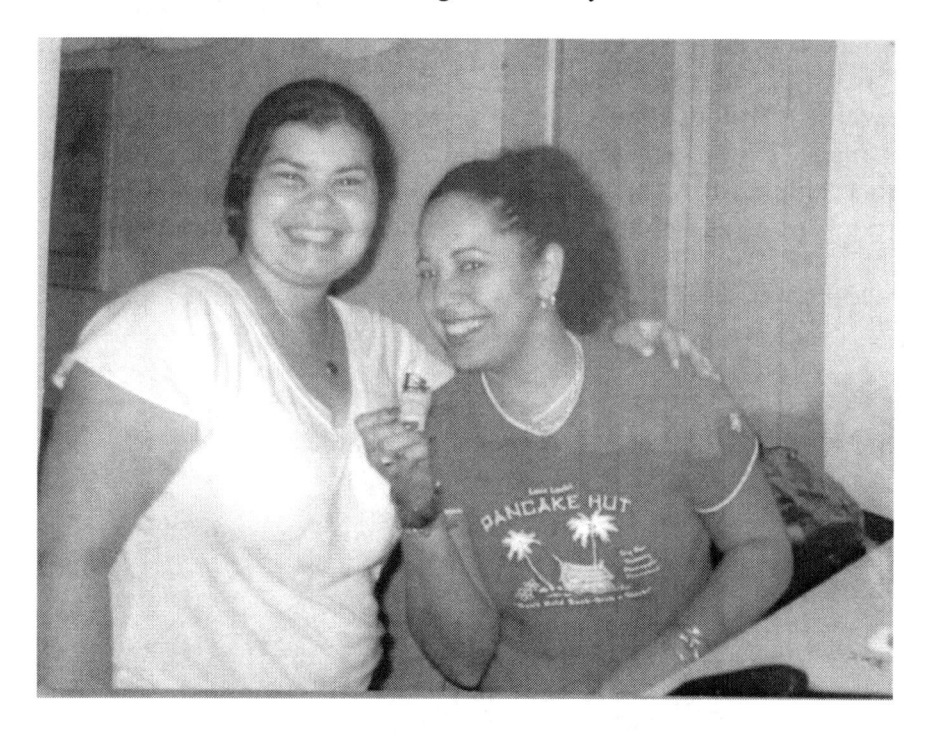

One step at a time. But perhaps most of all, find the right people to hang out with. Surround yourself with like-minded people.

Wayne Vandenlangenberg

Seven Hundred Pounds

Recently, I ran into someone who was a schoolmate of mine in grade school more than forty years ago. I say school "mate" but that's not exactly accurate. In fact, he was my chief tormentor. He bullied me horribly. I was very obese and he used to chase me up and down the stairs, delighting in the huge effort it was for me to escape his threats. But now, in Walmart more than four decades later, he was defensive. He also looked as if he were at least 75 pounds heavier than me. Things change, and for me, that change took me most of the four decades. It wasn't until I was literally about to die that I finally let go and dealt with the situation, a situation that began way back.

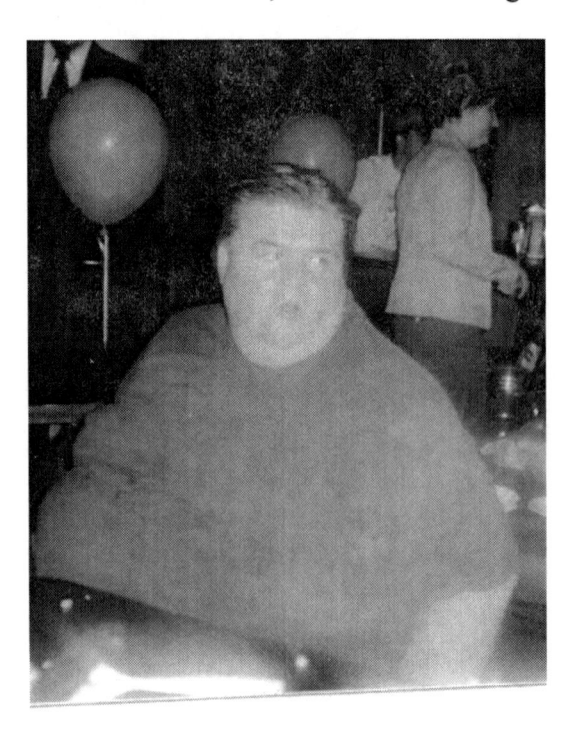

My early schooldays were very rough. I was the oldest of three brothers and a sister, and we lived with our parents just north of Green Bay, in Wisconsin. For whatever reason I was a huge kid. My father was actually tall and thin and although my mother gained weight after delivering each of her children, she wasn't morbidly obese like me. I weighed more than 200 pounds in elementary school, and I was miserable. I was always four paces behind everyone else -- and not just in the Hell that was known as the gym.

In the gym, I was always last in everything. One time, I heard another of my fellow students say to the gym teacher as I struggled to finish a run, "Why does he even bother?" To be honest, I was wondering that myself. There were absolutely no clothes that fit me. I had to wear outsized men's clothes. And as bad as they looked, I hated taking them off for gym even more. That's when the bullies would taunt me and snap towels at me. I was a big and easy target. I actually was afraid to go to school. I couldn't climb trees like the other kids. I couldn't do anything like the other kids. I was beaten up, humiliated and shamed every day at school. I felt like the biggest loser.

At home, my parents couldn't understand it. No one in my extended family was obese. In fact, they were all pretty fit, active and into sports. I felt as if I was an embarrassment to my entire family. When I expressed about one per cent of my torment to my parents they just told me I should "make more effort" and "just get along." My mom did join Weight Watchers at that time, and she did well. In fact, she looked fabulous. But she never took me, and I honestly don't know how much of her experience informed her efforts to help me.

My mother's approach to my weight was to give me small portions for my meals, and make me nasty lunches to take to school -- a little cheese, fruit and some milk. I often tried to trade with the other kids, but there were no takers. It didn't help that I went to a fairly small school, but even if it were ten times the size, I don't think I would have got any takers -- for anything.

My response to this enforced caloric restriction was to become the sneakiest food thief in Wisconsin, if not the entire Midwest. I found clever ways to steal food and great places to hide it --- like in my belly. Of course, there were sodas and snacks for my thinner siblings, so I always had plenty of choice and lots of opportunities. Sneaking food was my proudest accomplishment. But I still cried myself to sleep every night and hated waking up in the morning. Another day of torment.

Almost fifty years later, I talk at schools about my experiences, and I can relate to the stories that I hear. Recently, I was at a school where a young girl had just committed suicide after being bullied and tormented. "There but the grace of God go I."

The bullying continued all the way through my school career. I didn't know how to fight back or even that I should. I was so disconnected, which is painful in high school. I had very few friends. Even the nerdy kids didn't hang out with me. And I certainly wasn't getting any female attention. One time I plucked up enough courage to ask a girl to dance, and she laughed in my face. I was called about every name you can imagine from 'Chunky Monkey' to 'Fatso' and a lot of things in between.

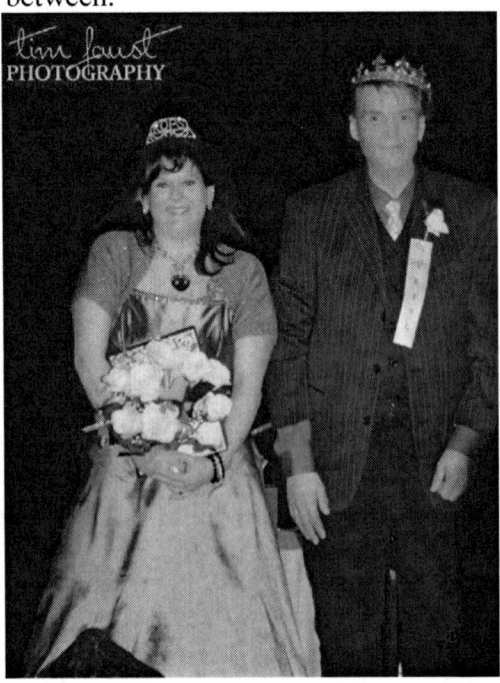

My high school was just three blocks away so I walked from home. I'm not sure I would have fit on the bus seat. I was well over 300 pounds. The school also had four floors, and it was very difficult for me to climb the stairs. Honestly, the only motivation was to get away from the tormentors who were snapping at my heels. As you might imagine, most of my time in class was spent watching the clock wind down, and plotting my escape. It was distracting. And on top of that my self-esteem was non-existent. I am amazed; I actually was a C student.

The only pleasure in my life was eating. I ate food I had hidden under my bed, in closets, and even in the garage. Even when I tried, I was betrayed by my corpulence. In High School, in an attempt to find some sort of place for myself, I turned to theater. I actually was in line for a good role in 'Man for All Seasons.' But this, too, turned out to be the theater of the absurd. The play is a period piece that requires some relatively expensive costumes. Mine would have to be custom made. They asked me whether I would want to be the stagehand in charge of lighting instead. It didn't matter. I still felt as if there was no recourse, and that I was a distant outcast flung far from the normal world.

It wasn't just the theater costumes that were a problem. Weighing more than 350 pounds, the only clothes that fit me were oversize men's golf gear. I graduated from high school without ever having a date, or so much as a cute conversation with a girl, let alone a conversation with a cute girl.

Given my school experience it's hardly any surprise that I chose not to pursue a college career. Naturally, perhaps, I gravitated to where I felt most comfortable, or actually the only place where I found any comfort at all. I quickly found a job in the food industry. My first job was at a restaurant, delivering pizzas. The owner allowed us to help ourselves to food while we worked, but I don't think he had my portions in mind when he created that policy. The amount of food I sneaked into my car and ate while on the job must have negatively impacted his bottom line while simultaneously increasing mine. It was the perfect job.

Things were picking up in my social life, too, or so I thought. I met a girl who was also plus size, which I thought was a plus, especially as I now weighed over 450 pounds. She was the first girl ever to give me any attention, and I loved it. All my siblings were getting married so I thought it would be a good idea if we did, too. It wasn't a good idea. We had fun while we were courting in those few months -- who doesn't? But the main course didn't live up to the appetizer. Nonetheless, it wasn't for lack of effort on my part.

In the year before we married, I lost 150 pounds. I basically went on a starvation diet. My pants size went down to a 42! I could actually buy regular clothes. I was walking regularly and not struggling. When the wedding came around I enjoyed being in the spotlight. It was the first time. I weighed about 300, as did my wife and were both about the same height -- six feet tall.

We were married for six years. As the euphoria and excitement of our initial relationship declined, my weight increased again. I was back into my old habits. Two years after our divorce I was back working at Hardee's. The restaurant chain provides employees with a uniform, but they didn't have one that fit me. I weighed over 400 pounds. I had to buy my own 'uniform.'

Laurie was the manager where I worked, and we didn't hit it off initially. But soon we had more than a friendship going. There was something about our relationship that I simply had a hard time accepting. I was untrusting, I guess. But Laurie told me that my weight wasn't important to her. Seriously? How could that be? She insisted it was me that she cared about, not my pants size.

Now I had a woman who loved me, and she didn't care how much I weighed. That seemed like the best of both worlds. So, I continued to indulge. Later, a nutritionist told me that I was eating thirteen thousand calories a day. 13,000 calories a day, on average.

By the time our wedding day rolled around, I was rolling around. I weighed 470 pounds, and my pants size was now up to a 64. I couldn't find a wedding suit. There was nothing for my size. And there was Laurie, all five feet and 190 pounds of her.

One of the interesting things about my eating at this time is that no matter how much I ate; I never felt full. I don't think I have ever felt full. I am told that the stomach stretch is what turns off appetite and sends signals to the brain to stop eating. I honestly don't think that until very recently I had that mechanism working in my guts. What was always there was the fear that I wasn't getting enough food.

Meanwhile, I left the food business, at least officially. I got a job as a taxi driver. This allowed me the freedom to go to every fast-food place, not just one. I drove around in between fares, ordering huge amounts of food. When I ordered, for example, ten cheeseburgers, I ordered them with different variations to make it look like I was buying for a team of people not just me. And, of course, it wasn't just the burgers; it was the sodas and fries, too. Then I would go home and cook an evening meal -- or seven. I cooked mostly high carb dinners, like pasta and pizza. Laurie ate a sensible portion, and I had the rest.

In the ensuing years, it got worse, if that's possible. I was regularly having thirty sodas a day. I could eat five gallons of ice-cream in three servings. I would eat countless bags of chips. I ate, I sat in front of the TV, planned the next day's feast and ate some more. I had no life outside of the taxicab. I didn't fit in any seats. I actually had to pay people to take my wife to the movies. I had a couple of pairs of very oversized shirts and pants at $70 each. I was isolated, watching the world -- and my life -- go by. How long could it go on like this?

It was the day after Thanksgiving in 2007. I felt dizzy and nauseated, which was unusual for me. I thought I was in okay health. Admittedly, I didn't go to doctors because I knew what they would tell me -- you need to lose weight. But on this day, I didn't feel good at all.

When I got to the clinic, they sent me immediately to the hospital. They frantically called an ambulance, which quickly arrived, but I didn't fit on the gurney. When I got to the hospital, I was code blue. My oxygen levels were dropping dangerously low. My breathing was at 39% capacity. I had pneumonia. There was fluid all around my organs. I was drowning from the inside out. I weighed more than 700 pounds. They told Laurie I wasn't going to make it.

I don't remember any of that. I fell into a coma. So, I don't recall the procedure that removed 80 pounds of fluid from my body in the first 48 hours in the intensive care unit.

I was in a coma for eleven days. There is only one thing that I can recall during that time.

I had been very close to my father's mother. She was probably the most encouraging and loving towards me of my whole family. She died eleven years earlier. But now, during my coma, I saw her again.

She looked young and was surrounded by light. I felt that special bond again. She spoke five words to me.

"You need to go back," she said softly.

When I came out of my coma, I didn't recognize my crying mom or my tearful wife at first. It didn't help that I had all sorts of tubes in me, including one in my trachea, which meant I could not talk. For quite a while, I had to communicate by writing short notes. I was in intensive care for 31 days. I had a speech therapist to help me get the right sounds out of my mouth and an eating therapist to help me get food into it. Unfortunately, I needed a physical therapist, but I didn't get one. I actually didn't get out of the bed for the entire 64 days I was in the hospital.

When I left the hospital, I left in a wheelchair. Being bedridden for two months wasn't good for me or my muscles. And disappointingly, my weight hadn't dropped much, apart for the 80 pounds of fluid that was removed in those first forty-eight hours.

I'd like to tell you that my brush with death made all the difference to me. I'd like to tell you that seeing my grandmother and having a near-death experience, if that's what it was, helped me see the light. But none of that happened, at least not immediately.

For the next six months, I returned to my old habits. There was one big difference, however. Laurie was losing her patience with me. The way I had been eating was no longer acceptable to her. What this meant, of course, was a return to sneaking food. I'd be home earlier than she, and cook myself all manners of things. She was unsuspecting and watched me eat a regular meal when she got home, not knowing that I had already eaten a significant amount prior to her arrival.

Then in June, the 24th to be exact, it happened. As you have read, I have spent a lot of the days of my life watching TV. I happen to be a big Days of Our Lives fan, especially of Alison Sweeney. On June 24, 2008, I was channel surfing and saw Alison on a new show. She was hosting a show called The Biggest Loser. I didn't know much about the show, but I continued watching so I could see Alison. During the show, there was an advertisement for LA Weight Loss centers. I checked out the local franchise and made an appointment. I was ready. Finally.

At L.A. Weight Loss, I was interviewed by a very compassionate young lady, appropriately named Wendy. I'm not sure she had ever seen someone who weighed 600 pounds before. Having spoken with her for a while, she sat back in her chair and said, "I'm sorry, there's nothing we can do for you."

I broke down. I was finally ready to let my guard down and deal with my huge problem and there was nothing she could do for me?

Sensing my frustration and the inherent absurdity of turning away a 600 pound man who had just decided to seek help, Wendy picked up the phone and called the corporate office. God bless her! She pleaded my case. I waited to hear the verdict.

"Okay," she said, "If you can get two doctors to agree to medically supervise you, we'll accept you into the program."

I breathed a huge sigh of relief. I'm not sure but having been so close to being turned away might have actually helped me. I had been given a last chance at my last chance. I was immediately able to get two local doctors to agree to cover me medically, and I was on my way.

I was given a menu of controlled food items and calorie limits. I followed it religiously without much of a problem. I finally faced up to the fact of where I was heading; a spectacle in a double casket in a funeral home.

On my first weigh-in, I lost 19 pounds. By November, almost a year after that fateful trip to the hospital, I was down 94 pounds.

Then disaster struck. The LA Weight Loss Center I was going to, closed its doors. I was devastated. I was doing so well and had developed a great relationship with them. And now they were gone.

Of course, I drowned my sorrows the only way I know how and promptly regained sixty pounds. But by the New Year, I had found another program and was back on track.

I cut out processed foods, but mostly the high glycemic carbs, red meat and soda. When I went to the store, I avoided the center aisle where most of that food is. I just didn't want to go near it.

Now I was focused and with Laurie's support, I was on my way. I averaged a loss of four pounds a week. By the end of the year, I was down 200 pounds. Of course, I was still an obese 450 pounds, but at least I was going in the right direction. Then I could see a difference in my 'before' and 'after' photos. Within a few short weeks, I was out of my wheelchair and using a walker. It wasn't too long before I was down to just using a cane. Then, I started walking. My goal was five miles a day, and I did that pretty much every day even if it took me two or three trips to get the mileage in.

I never deviated from the plan. I ate sensibly, and I walked. I felt good, better than I ever have. I started living life again instead of watching it go by. I kept losing at a good rate so that by the end of 2010, I had lost another 200 pounds. At my highest, my shirt size had been a 6x, now it was a medium. My pants had been an 89, now they were a 31. I loved shopping for clothes! For the first time in my life, I could actually buy regular clothes.

The word got out about my four hundred-pound weight loss, and I was invited on to the set of the Biggest Loser where I actually met Alison Sweeney. It was one of the best days of my life! I weighed 256 pounds. But it didn't stop there. I was then invited on to the Jay Leno show.

Jay was amazing. He actually sat in my dressing room, and we talked about life, Wisconsin and the Green Bay Packers for a long time. He really put me at my ease. He made sure that Laurie was flown out to Hollywood to be with me. By this time, Laurie had lost a few pounds, too. Well, almost 60.

Jay had encouraged me to relax, be myself and "make it real." He did a great job. When he told the audience that my wife and I had met at Hardee's where we both worked, he turned to me and asked; "Did you make out by the fryer?"

Having been well prepared by the wonderful Mr. Leno I didn't miss a beat.

"No, we actually did that in the freezer."

My fifteen minutes of fame -- I think it was thirteen minutes actually -- went well. Later, I was on Access Hollywood.

Then I started to regain the weight and honestly panic a bit. So I decided to join a local weight loss support group --TOPS. When I walked through those doors on July 11th 2012, I was looking for help. I knew of the group from a few of members in and around my area. I was actually afraid to step on the scale my first day. I knew I had gained some back due to stress in my life-- which goes to show you I am human-- and needed a support group to get back on track.

I stepped on the scale, and it topped 302. I had not been in the 300's for a year at best. Well, I knew right then and there; I was going to join and win this battle and reach my goal. I was close to my goal --

a small matter of eighty pounds or so to go -- and I knew with their support, I would get there. In my first six months I lost 87 pounds, and the following year I lost my last 6 pounds. I reached my goal of 210 and was named Wisconsin State King -- the male TOPS member in the state, who had lost the most weight in the year -- for 2013.

What I have learned is everyone needs help to win the obesity battle. I thought I could do it on my own, and I found out I did indeed need the accountability. With that again in my life, I was successful in reaching that final goal, a goal I never thought would happen. My group, which I call family now, are like mothers, brothers and sisters to me. I am forever grateful they opened not just their doors to me but their hearts, too.

I have been at a healthy weight for three years. My BMI was 88, now it's 19.2; helped a bit by the removal of more than 22 pounds of skin in 2013.

I've adapted. I still go to fast-food places, but I have the chicken without the bun, and fruit rather than fries. I swim three or four times a week and also use a treadmill. I am very fortunate in that neither diabetes nor high cholesterol have never been a problem. I work at the airport preparing food, but it doesn't bother me. Generally, I just make myself a small salad and that is sufficient.

My almost five hundred-pound weight loss -- from my highest weight going into the hospital -- not to mention my television appearances, have earned me some notoriety. I have used it to hit the road and spread the word. I go to schools, health fairs, and weight loss groups. If I can change just one person, then all the talks and the travel will be well worth it.

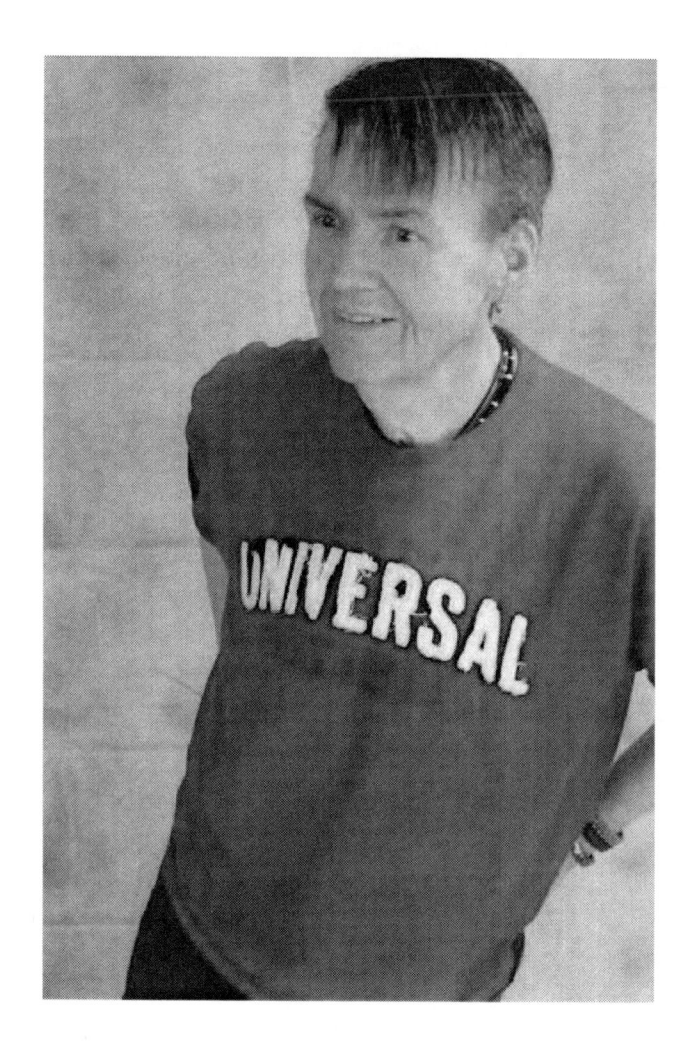

My message is simple.

Love yourself.

For too long, I was still that bullied kid in an adult body. I was hurt, angry, and lost. Now, I have found inner peace. I have no resentment. I forgive the bullies and tormentors, and I forgive myself.

There's no magic unless loving yourself is magic. And sometimes it is.

There is one other ingredient; however, that you need.

I couldn't have done this without my wonderful wife. She took our wedding vows seriously. When I was sick, she nursed me. She changed my tubes; she cleaned me up; she nurtured me. She loved me unconditionally and without her, I'm not sure I would have ever got to the point of caring about myself. She encouraged me; she reminded me when I might have strayed. 90% of my progress is down to her.

I truly believe that I do not need the food and eating the way I did before. I finally faced my demons.

It took me a long time, but I finally have found myself.

Karl Steeves

Build Your Body to Build Your Self

I am the only child of military parents. I was born in San Diego and moved to Jacksonville at the age of 7. My dad was in the Navy, and my mom was actually a Navy reservist when I was born. The Navy plays a large part in my story.

My parents were into fitness. Dad did a lot of triathlons. He was a weight lifter, and his interest in that activity has had a huge influence in my life. My mom was also into fitness. She is 5'1" tall and weighs about 100 pounds. She is holistic expert and it often seemed to me that she was waging a single-handed battle against modern medicine! She can be tough. She absolutely would not let me eat any candy of any sort when I was a child, with the result that I have always craved it. I was home-schooled until the age of twelve.

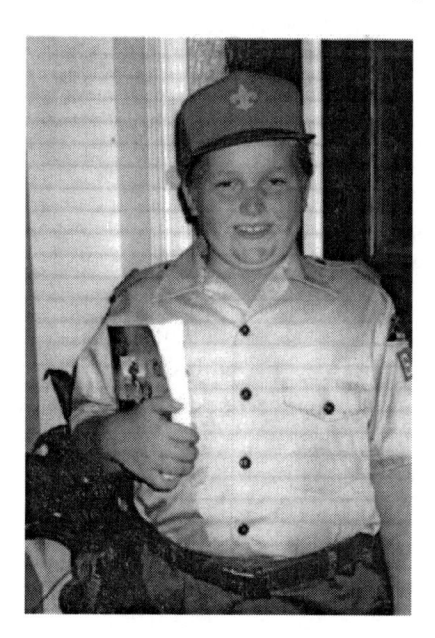

All my grandparents gained weight as they aged. (That's not for me. I want to be doing squats and having sex when I'm 90 -- 'though not necessarily at the same time.) I had a stocky disposition as a child. I was a chubby baby and remained overweight until my teen years. I was teased and bullied when I did go to school. The girls avoided me, and the boys called me "fat ass." My social skills weren't great, and I was a nerdy kid. A frustrated, nerdy kid.

But then, as I entered my teen years, I had a growth spurt and also started going to the gym. If the truth be told, I was tired of being fat, and everything that went along with it.

A history as a fat, introverted, and socially awkward kid; however, is hard to overcome. From the onset of youth, the images of masculinity, toned physiques, six-pack abs and arms like pythons are ingrained into our minds and become the standard by which looks are judged by. I was never blessed with genetics for looks or a body that denounces fat. Instead, I was blessed with an average face and a torso that screams in delight when pie and pizza are thrown down the gullet.

In high school, despite my disadvantages, I tried to become athletic and played every sport imaginable but especially baseball. I also went on a sort of Paleo diet and gave up processed food.

I came to see the gym as my sanctuary, a place where I felt in control and where the results were dependent entirely on me. The scale doesn't lie. I saw fitness as both an outlet and a stress manager. I liked the fact that I dictated what happened in the gym. I guess it was also a reflection of my mental state at the time that I took an interest in the science of fear. At school, I was good at the subjects I was interested in, everything else I just mailed in.

By the time I was fourteen I was playing football and hanging out with the cooler kids. My confidence increased, and I started to get some female attention. I was 5'9" and weighed 140.

Through the high school years, I was in good shape and played sports. My dad subscribed to body-building magazines, and I started to take an interest in that activity, too. My dad was supportive and showed me the basics of lifting, and we could often be seen working out together in our garage. It turns out that I have the right physique for a weight lifter as I have very strong legs. It wasn't long before I could dead-lift 300 pounds.

After graduating from high school, I wasn't sure what I wanted to do. So, naturally, I joined the Navy. Three years later, I was ripped! I had done a lot of lifting, and it was doing me good. I was very specifically exercising for the purpose of body-building. My confidence was high, and my social skills were improving. I was getting a lot of female attention.

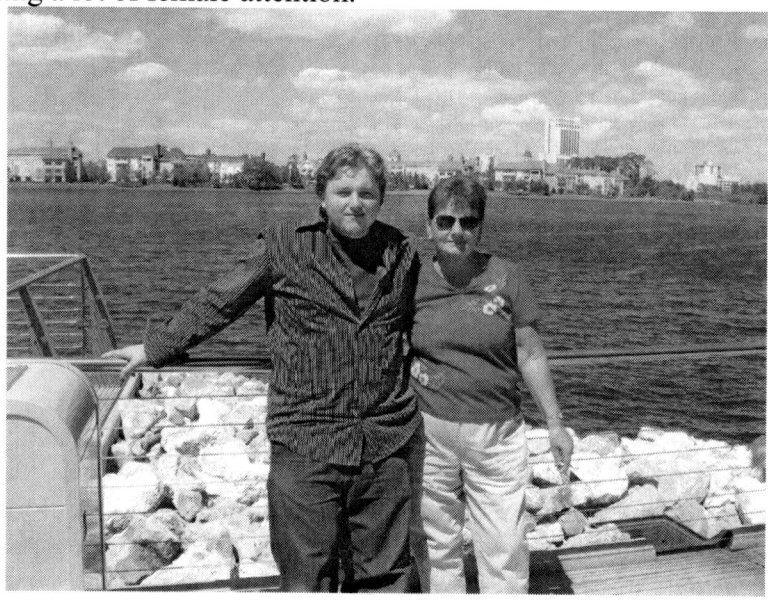

Despite these occasional successes, however, I had been conditioned to see myself as fat, out of place, awkward and unaccepted. Over the years, as I flirted with the idea of sports, lifting, dieting and physique change, at best it felt good but at worst, when the motivation dried up, and I was back to square one, I felt even angrier at myself.

This is what happened after I had been in the Navy for a while. For some reason, I lost interest. I'm not sure what happened, but in any event when I was deployed to Iraq, I was a pudgy 230. When I returned from Iraq, I had lost about twenty-five pounds and was lifting again. I could bench-press 315 pounds. When I got back stateside the Navy gave me a physical. They used some advanced measure of body fat, which claimed I was 24% body fat. This didn't make sense to me. A caliper measure around the same time had my body fat at 13%. Nonetheless, I was designated as fat and was assigned to the 'fat program,' which meant working out three times a week. My oppositional self really came out, and all my motivation disappeared. My weight increased to 240. Within six months I was discharged, honorably but fat.

I drifted. I got a variety of jobs; working in a hotel and a liquor store, I even got licensed as a heating and air conditioning engineer. I didn't care. I did have a girlfriend for a while but even that wasn't going anywhere. I was lost.

I ended back on my mom's couch. She and my dad had been divorced for a few years at this point. I couldn't find work. I just hung out, read fantasy books and played video games. I didn't want to face the truth.

My eureka moment came when I was preparing to go to a wine-tasting event with my girlfriend.

I wanted to look good and wear some nice clothes for a change. I had some cool clothes in my wardrobe. In fact, some of them used to be baggy on me, but now I could barely fit into them. When I took a really good look in the mirror, I was shocked. My stomach was hanging out; my face appeared fat, and I looked terrible. I had to discard the cool clothes and put on the baggiest shirt I could find. That night, I really didn't want to venture out in public.

"I'm fat. I can't let people see me like this," I said to my girlfriend.

Suddenly, it struck me that my weight and fitness had to become my priority again.

It was almost as if some sensible, responsible person stepped out of me. He said, "You're a sad, disgusting being."

My girlfriend Jess said, "Come on, you're not that bad."

But she was being an enabler. I *was* that bad.

There was a gym just down the road, and I quickly rejoined and threw myself back into fitness. It was the spring of 2008. I would go every day and work on different muscle groups as well as doing cardio. Monday, it was chest, Tuesday, legs, Wednesday, back and so on.

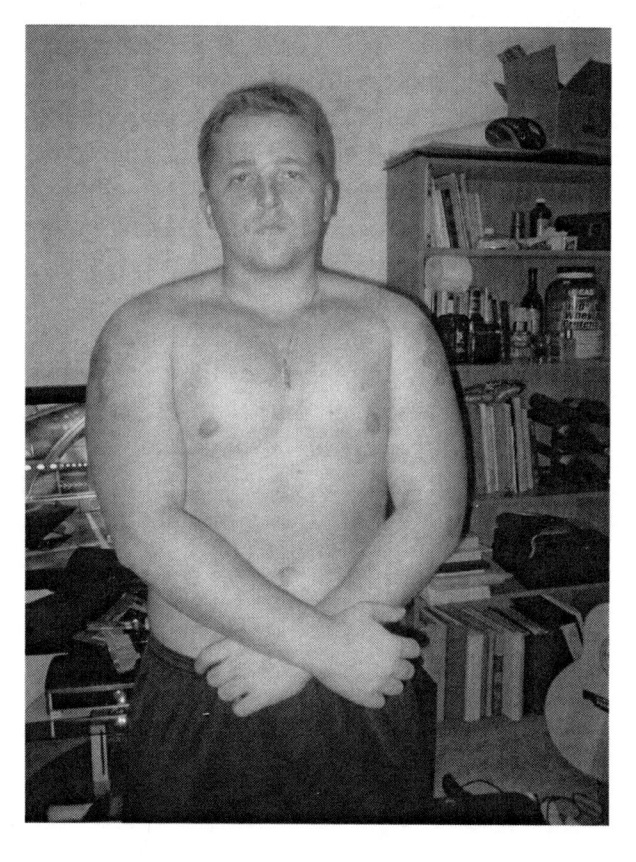

Gradually, I was finding my way back. I was also doing lots of research on fitness and lifting, but that didn't prevent me from overdoing some exercises and occasionally burning out. Overall, however, my mood lifted. My energy increased, and my confidence started to return.

In a couple of months, by the summer of 2008, I got a contract job in Kuwait. The job involved up-fitting vehicles to make them more secure. This involved inserting plates of steel in the undercarriage, the doors, and other different vulnerable parts of the car.

It was a really rewarding job. I honestly believe that this company saved lives, and I was helping them. I worked incredibly hard. I was working at least 12 hours a day, up-fitting numerous vehicles and lifting pieces of steel, some of which weighed two hundred pounds. Some of the older workers told me not to work so hard. "You'll hurt yourself," they warned.

On top of the workload, I was also going to the gym, lifting weights, and doing cardio. Some of the people at the gym were also concerned I was going to hurt myself or do something to my back, but I was loving it. It also helped that I was making great money.

The more I worked out, the healthier I felt, the better I slept, the easier it became to work out more. I dropped 20 pounds very quickly. My body was really the perfect fit for the physical labor I was doing. It soon became that fitness was a way of life. It was implicit. I admit I was driven. I had a huge chip on my shoulder. I wanted to prove all my detractors -- from the bullies in school, to the doubters in the Navy -- that they were wrong about me.

I turned to CrossFit for about 18 months. I was pushing myself to the limit and competing in lifting and other events, just for fun. By 2011, I had dropped another 30 pounds and was down to around 200.

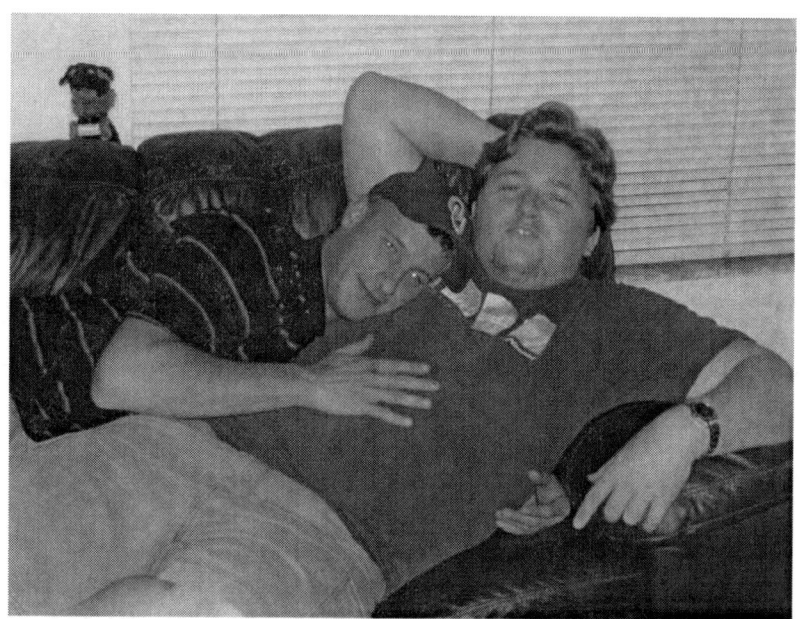

During this time, I had a thought about how I could really prove the detractors wrong. I obsessed about a particular plan to the point where it became a stated goal. After weeks of obsessing, I was sure what I wanted to do.

I wanted to join the Navy SEALs.

I started preparing myself for the challenge. I found out that I had until I was thirty years old to make it.

I researched what was required to become a SEAL. I spent hours watching videos and researching BUDS -- the intense SEALs training course. I made getting into BUDS and becoming a SEAL my whole life.

I developed a punishing schedule of heavy compound movements, like squats to develop muscle, sprints, conditioning swimming and ultra-long runs. I could dead-lift 600 pounds. I ran 4 miles in under 32 minutes. Although real strength takes years to develop, cardio conditioning develops very quickly. I was building a lot of muscle. Actually, a lot of my calorie intake went toward that goal.

Remember, the more muscle you have, the higher your metabolism because muscle burns a lot more than fat.

I was pumped, literally and metaphorically. I was ultra-disciplined in my diet. I really fought the cravings, especially for pizza. I was driven by higher goals. I knew that as a SEAL I could not accept being mediocre. I had to stay ultra-competitive, or I wouldn't make it through BUDS. I know that if you stop growing you start dying. I knew I had to get it right the first time, every time. I was the quintessential alpha male.

I had put in my application for BUDS through the SEALs. In the spring of 2013, I got the word.

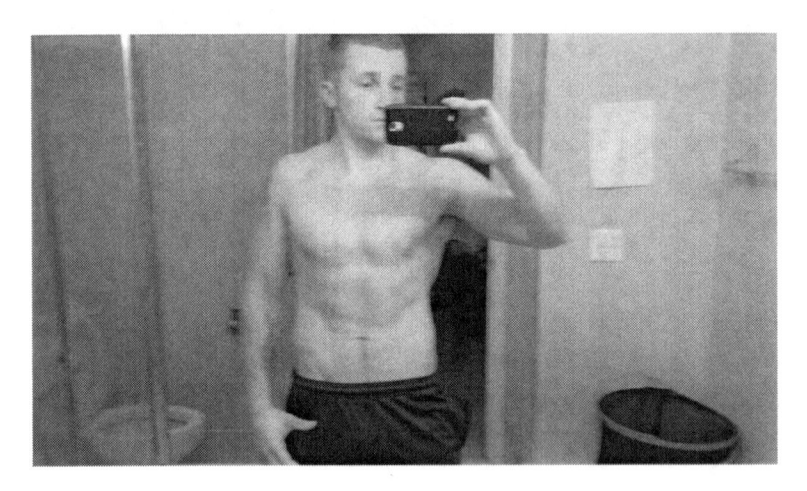

My application didn't just have to go through the SEALs it had to go through the Navy, too. And, given my previous service record, and especially the fat issue just prior to my discharge, they wouldn't accept me. My dream disappeared in a flash.

The day I got the news, I drank half a bottle of scotch, and I'm not normally a drinker. Even now, I can't watch SEALS videos or movies; it's simply too depressing.

With my SEALs dream over, I had to change my focus. I soon made it my number-one goal to become a world-class weight lifter. I knew I would need at least two years of practice and development to be a legitimate, competitive lifter rather than an average fat lifter. I cut back on the cardio, and gradually my physique changed.

Honestly, the notion of being a world-class lifter is a nice fantasy. Here's really how I have come to view working-out and what it means to me.

Vanity is biologically driven, socially approved, and narcissistically reinforced. Many work out in order to achieve this goal: I am one of them. However, I do not allow the pursuit of fleeting aesthetic fame to drive my own purpose, nor do I derive meaning from shallow fruitless endeavors culminated by thousands of crunches and bicep curls. Instead, I accept the fate for what it is; a shallow, fleeting, and selfish bout of identity that once achieved, will be put aside with a smile while more meaningful pursuits turn from dreams into reality.

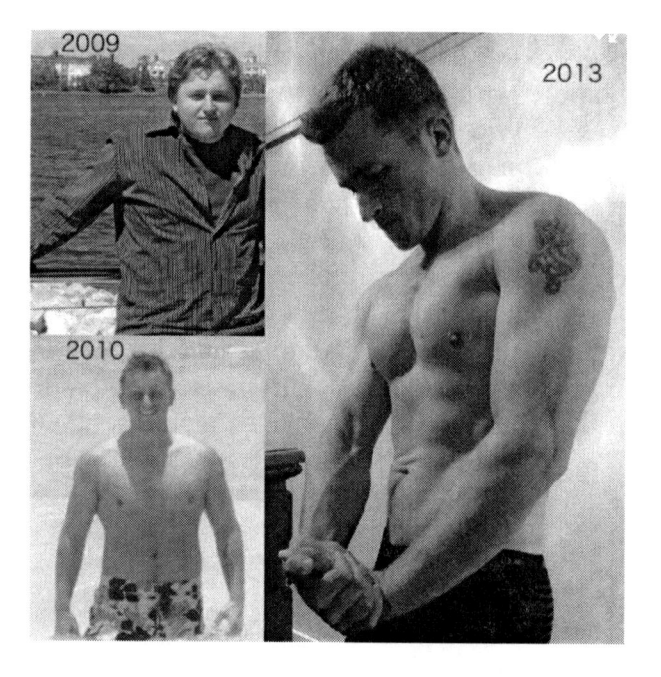

As I stated above, initially I was one of the masses who want a body that will elicit gawks and stares and a bit of inner doubt to those not yet on my level. This is a natural desire born out of the want of something I've never had, and honestly, never thought possible. It, however, does not define me, nor does it give me the energy to devote my free time to so many hours grueling away. I think the aesthetics is a by-product of a greater goal, and not the end goal in and of itself.

I view my lifting as a euphoric time when all else is turned off, nothing matters, my mind is in a nirvana, and I can see -- no, feel -- the tangible results of my work and efforts. I have grown fascinated with the human body. It is the most amazing machine this planet has ever seen, each one bearing many similarities but each unique in its own right. I strive to push my body in an effort to realize what it is capable of doing. I was never born the strongest, fastest, quickest or most athletic, but what I have is a drive that stems from the intrinsic motivation of never being satisfied and the fear of stagnation.

The looks I get are my external motivation, my lifts are internal. I don't lift to impress others; I don't try beating a swim or run time to blast the results to my friends to show I am better than them; I train because each time I beat an old distance, lift more weight, or learn a new movement. I have proven to myself that I have become better; I have succeeded; I am one step closer to discovering the absolute best that I can produce. For me, there is no better reason, no more motivation is needed. I thoroughly enjoy what I do, and through lifting I have discovered ways of improving many other aspects of my life. I am home at the gym, running sprints in the park; hiking trails or swimming in the ocean. I am in tune with my body, and in the same respects with my mind. I have discovered a deep longing for betterment, and the better I become the more I want to achieve.

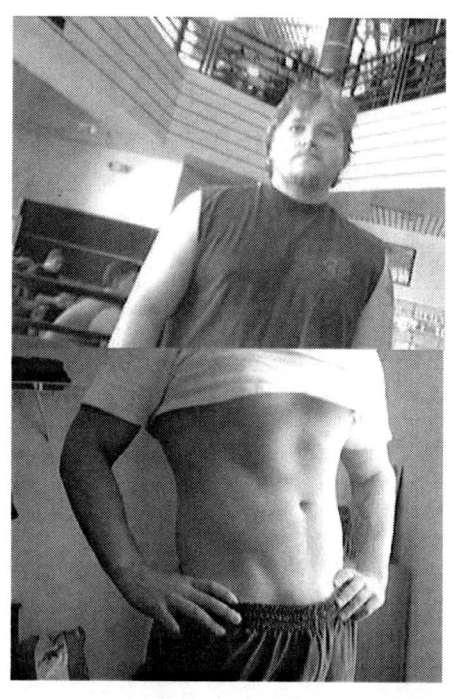

I lift because it is the one venue where I control the outcome, I make and pursue my own challenges, and I determine if my outcome is satisfactory. I long for those brief moments when all that matters is the next rep, the next jump, pushing my time faster. In lieu of deriving satisfaction from unhealthy vices, I gain my euphoria from strengthening and pushing my body. Really, I have no dreams of frivolous fame and fortune. I am not an elite athlete, and when I die, no one will remember how many times I could dead-lift 500lbs at some random gym. But that is irrelevant, for it matters to my mind and my person, for I do this for me and no one else. Sure, I'd love to prove wrong, the people who doubted and ridiculed me, but like the aesthetics they're an afterthought, nothing more than the side of ketchup to my burger and fries. I push myself to achieve the point where all else can wait, where I can stop thinking about what I'm going to accomplish in my life, why I am here, what stresses are hounding me today. I seek out, even if for a few fleeting seconds, that moment of blissful peace where I am one. And that mindset has allowed me to appreciate my body, and it has responded. It is in great shape, but that is just the bi-product.

Yes, as you can tell I am a completely different person than I was three years ago. There are some important lessons that I have learned along the way that I want to share with you.

When you're passionate about a goal, don't ever give up.

There are a lot of recommendations and advice out there about everything. Everyone is different. Do what is right for you, what works for you.

Don't have tempting food around. I do three grocery shops a week and buy a little at a time so that there's not too much around the house. Your home is not a food bank. If there's food around you're going to eat it.

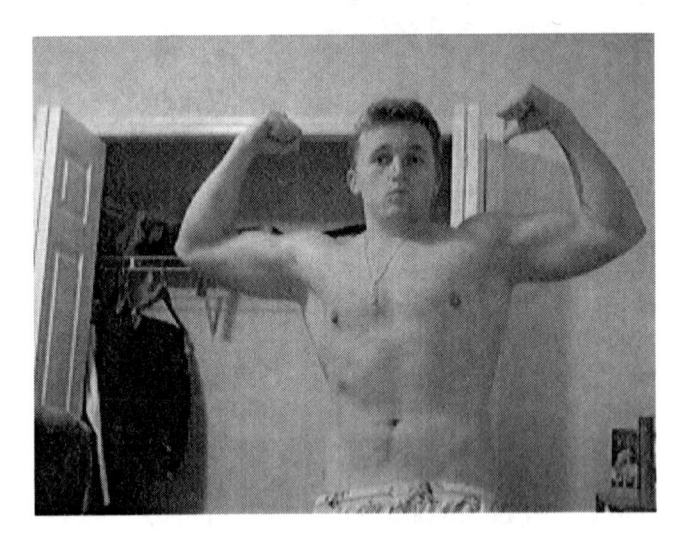

You can train yourself to eat vegetables! We're biologically meant to eat veggies.
I've learned to love them. I started with Romaine lettuce. I now have raw kale with almonds as a morning snack. It's delicious. It used to take me three weeks to go through a bag, now it's gone in two days! I also have a lot of high-fiber grains, eggs and fruit. Nutritional balance matters and macronutrient requirement are different for everyone.

You have to build in some "treats". You can't be restrictive all the time. You need to have some fun days. I call them 'Fat Karl' days. I love chocolate. I say to myself 'I promise I won't eat it all', but I have to be honest with myself.

Don't set yourself up for failure by being around the wrong food and the wrong people. Forget about the quick fix, that's the wrong expectation.

You need to have phases where the goal is to maintain weight, not lose it. Maintaining is much harder than losing. Maintenance doesn't just happen; you have to work at it -- all the time.

Be prepared to work hard. Some days I'm at the gym for five hours and need four thousand calories to repair my body. You need to strive to thrive.

Surround yourself with supportive people. My girlfriend Karla is very supportive. She doesn't nag me; she encourages me and makes me feel attractive. Warren, my best friend, is always pushing me on to greater challenges.

Appreciate your achievements and effort. There are kids at the gym that look up to me. At first, I dismissed it, but then I realized that I am at the pinnacle of fitness. I want to help and motivate people. Some of my Facebook buddies say that I inspire them.

Stay connected to your motivation. I've felt like a failure many times, and I don't want my detractors to be right. I'm terrified of being that fat guy again. Think long term. Think how you will be when you're older. You want to preserve your body. The body is a wonderful masterpiece, and I don't want to abuse it, and neither should you.

The harder you work, the easier it gets. Although I've had a few physical issues, for example, a torn rotator cuff, it has mostly gotten easier.

Physical fitness develops self-esteem. You're not just developing muscle; you're developing psychological endurance, too. And ladies, don't be afraid to lift weights. You won't get muscle bound, but you need to develop muscle mass to improve fitness and metabolism.

Meditation and similar relaxation techniques help you stay focus and keep things in perspective.

And finally, as someone who has been bullied and teased and knows the devastating effects that taunting can have on a person's self-esteem, I ask you this: Never be demeaning to someone. Not only does it hurt others, in the end the only one that looks stupid is you.

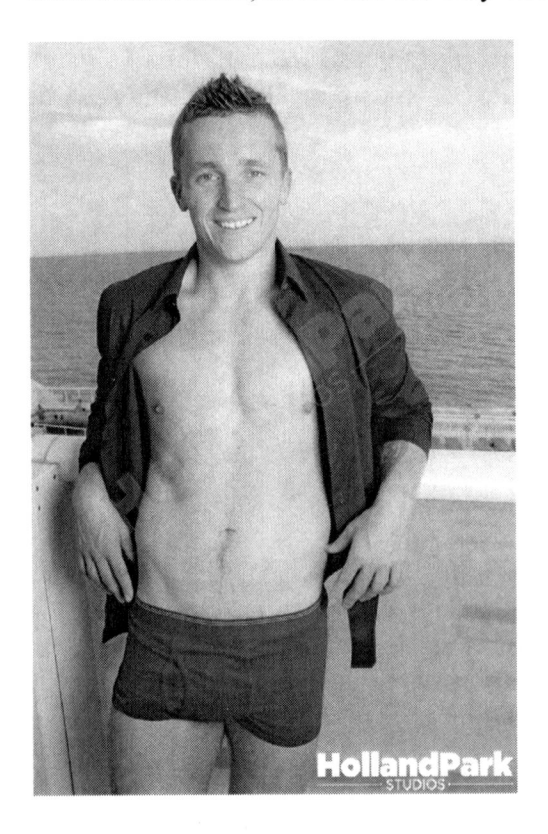

Dione Housden

Ten Per Cent at a Time

November 1992. It's confirmed. I am going on a trip to New York with my family. Great! I know I need to lose weight for this vacation. We are going to be very active, and I will never be able to keep up if I don't shed some weight. I know we will be walking a lot, all over the Big Apple, and I don't want to be the one to hold everyone else up.

I weighed 380 pounds and with some focus and dedication, I lost 60 pounds. I had a great time in New York, especially as I had lived on the West Coast my entire life. I came back from that vacation and promptly gained all the weight back -- and more.

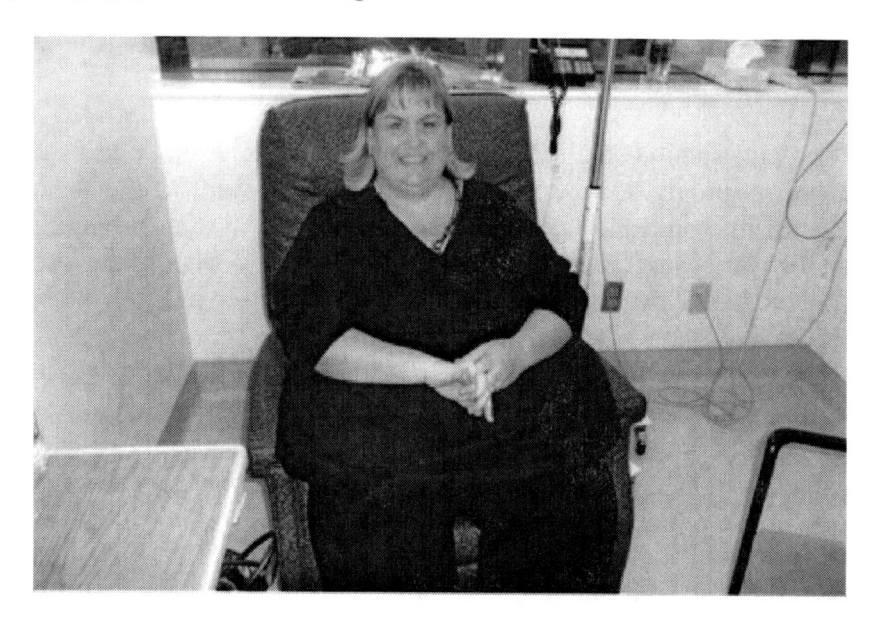

The problem was that I went on a diet, and I've learned the hard way that diets don't work. Despite my lofty scale numbers, it was my first serious attempt to lose weight. It was 10 years after getting married, a decade after really packing on the pounds.

Even though that time in 1992 was my first concerted weight loss effort, I feel as if I've been a diet my entire life. I honestly don't look overweight when I see photos from my childhood and adolescence. But I felt as if I was. I've wondered why, but I think there are two main reasons.

I did feel different. Part of that reason was that I was a very tall 5'9" at an early age, and I am always in the back row of those school photos. Looking back at those photos now, I don't see an overweight child. I was recently going through some of those photos with my mom. She looked at one of the pictures and said, "You look good in this photo." I replied, "It still wasn't good enough for you." She said, "You know you're right." I think it was an eye-opener for her. Maybe she was afraid and very concerned I would gain weight. Every parent wants their kids to fit in, and maybe my folks were just really afraid that I wouldn't. I was already the big girl -- as in tall. Mom didn't have a weight problem, but she did go to various groups and was careful about her eating.

My parents spent a small fortune taking me to clinics and putting me on special programs when I was young. I even went to the Schick program in Seattle. In case you haven't heard of it, that program is famous for using aversion therapy or electric shocks to treat addictive behavior. Here's a shock for you; it didn't work.

I was very active as a child. Kids back then had imaginations and if the sun was shining, we played outside. I was very energetic, no video games or computers or iTunes, just running around. Even after I gained weight, I remained very active -- cleaning house, doing yard work, etc., etc. I never stopped, still don't, there's always a lot to do.

When I was sixteen, my dad even promised me a car if I lost weight. When I look back, I only had 30 pounds to lose!! I wasn't the only one in my extended family who was overweight but everyone else only seemed to be fifteen pounds overweight. I was the outlier, especially as I got older.

As a result, I've done every single plan: Atkins, low-carb, hi-carb, NutriSystems, you name it - I've done it.

So, I went through my childhood and adolescence thinking that I was fat and feeling as if I was constantly monitored. I'm sure my parents' intentions were great, but the burden was heavy. Very heavy. My parents always seemed worried about food and what I was eating. Mom denies it. In her defense, my brother (older by seven years) was not overweight as a child, although he has gained some during his early retirement. Maybe I just interpreted her natural desire to do the best for me as monitoring and restriction.

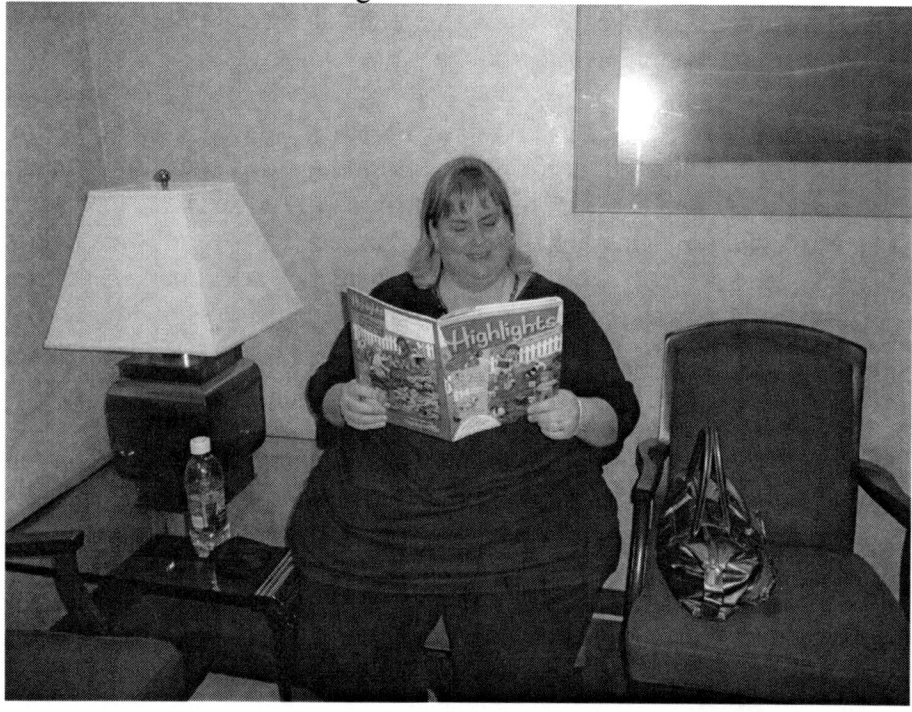

Perhaps it was a subconscious thing that I couldn't have identified or articulated when I was a child. But the fact is, for whatever reason, when I left home at twenty and got married, I promptly gained 100 pounds. Yes, the very first year of my marriage, I gained 100 pounds!

Liberated from whatever chains I imagined were at home, I went wild. I bought anything I wanted, and I wanted a lot.

I was in denial. It is odd. It's not until you see yourself in photos, do you have a good sense of how others see you. To me, I always looked exactly the same regardless of my weight. I did a double-take and had absolute mirror shock when I was 20 years old and saw a much fatter girl looking back at me. Where did she come from?

Within the next few years, I gained another 100 pounds. I still lived in the same area as my parents and I don't remember them commenting about my weight during this time. It was the voices in my own head who really knew, the ones doing a number on me. A number that eventually grew to 430.

So, yes, I went from 180 to 380 in 10 years. I thought about dieting every day. I started a diet every Monday, and was done every Tuesday. When I was two days into it, it seemed too hard, impossible, so I gave up. I've since learned that severely restrictive eating plans simply don't work. They are not sustainable, and you can't live that way. I know I can't live on boiled eggs for the rest of my life.

So, 10 years later, now married twenty years and weighing over 400 pounds, I was cleaning house one Saturday, and there's a knock on the door. I opened the door and saw a lovely lady standing there. She was smiling and looking very sociable. She said, "You don't know who I am?"

"No I don't," I replied, "Who are you?"

She happened to be a very good friend of mine, Mary. In fact, she actually introduced me to my husband -- and I still consider her a friend!! I simply didn't recognize her! She had lost so much weight; she was literally unrecognizable. When it dawned on me who she was, I grabbed her by the scruff of her neck and pulled her into the house, and I wasn't letting her go until she had given me the magic formula to her weight-loss success.

How did you do this?

She told me that she had used Slimfast. I, too, had tried it once before but given Mary's story, I thought it was time to do it again. So, I went out and bought a semi truck's worth of the product -- mostly bars and shakes. I had Slimfast for breakfast and lunch and then a regular, healthy dinner. I didn't want to cook for my husband and not eat it, too. We ate together at dinner; chicken, meat, fish with salad, mostly. I was extremely successful. I lost 160 pounds on my Slimfast program in about 15 months.

Then I hit a plateau and was concerned and frustrated. I asked all sorts of people how to get beyond it. Someone said I should go back to the way I was eating before for a while and then get back on the Slimfast. This would shock my body, and I would get going again, this person said. I liked that idea! So that's what I did.

I went back to my old eating habits. But, of course, I never did get back on Slimfast. I gained all that 160 pounds back... plus more. It seemed like it happened overnight, like I just woke up and was fat again. I really don't remember putting the weight back on. It's odd, but it was just there. 160 pounds just materialized. I'm honestly not sure how long it took, but it was probably about a year -- though it seemed like it was a week.

I was so frustrated. I gave up. Statistics weren't on my side.

I was 430 at my highest. I gave up on dieting. It obviously wasn't going to work. My glittering history of failure was no cause for optimism or hope. I gave up on my weight and focused on making myself happy. Everything else in my life was great, so I had plenty to live for and enjoy. I had a good job, a great marriage, a house, everything I wished for.

In 2007, in my mid-40s, I didn't go to doctors. I don't like them. I was overweight, so I didn't want to be embarrassed, and I didn't have any health problems that I knew of. I was on no medication and felt fine. My husband and parents, however, kept encouraging me to go.

"You're in your mid-40s you should make sure everything is okay, and you're not headed for some health issues," they said.

So, reluctantly I made an appointment, even though I felt it was a waste of time and money.

I went to the appointment very confident, almost cocky, and definitely rebellious. The thoughts were running in my head about the doctor and his staff. "They're going to be surprised at how healthy I am." "They're going to assume something is wrong with me but there won't be." "They're going to have to eat their words that fat people are unhealthy." Bring it on. Then, I can silence my parents once and for all and stop their silly, pointless, misguided scare tactics.

That day I found out I was lying. That day I found out I was dying.

By the time I left the doctor, there was so much wrong with me; I wasn't sure I'd make it to the car. I called my husband. I was sobbing, "I'm not going to make it home."

Every test score that was supposed to be high was low, and everything that was supposed to be low was high. I was a mess.

Cholesterol was sky high -- in orbit, actually. My blood pressure was so high that they had to give me some medication to take, right there and then, to prevent a stroke. There were nervous even to send me home.

But the biggest problem by far was the other news.

I was diabetic.

You need to know that I have always been terrified of needles. After they told me I was diabetic, all I could hear was ringing in my ears and the question resounding in my head, "How am I going to live the rest of my life stabbing myself with a needle?"

I couldn't wrap my head around it. It was a death sentence. I couldn't fathom it.

So, something had to be done about it. The doctor sat me down and said:

"You know, if you take off some of this weight, some of these problems might go away."

The exact words he said were absolutely critical. Can you tell which ones that had the most impact?

"If you take off **some** of this weight." He didn't say you have to take off all of your weight, just some of it.

That was a huge deal. He didn't come out and say you need to lose 200 pounds, just "some of this weight." Some of this weight was manageable. All of it? It would have been too daunting. Nobody loses 200 pounds. It would have seemed impossible.

Immediately after the visit, I researched everything I could. I had been looking up facts about nutrition, and I had read this article about the extreme benefits of losing just 10% of your body weight. I learned that many of the greatest advantages and health benefits occur with the first 10% of weight loss, apparently. Whether that's completely true or not, it made my task manageable. Could I lose 200 pounds? Not a chance. But I knew I could lose 40 pounds. And when you're 400 pounds, 40 pounds is really nothing.

I started working with a nutritionist, and she had me weigh and measure absolutely everything I put in my mouth. I mean everything. That was the hardest thing I ever did, but it helped saved my life. I also went to a diabetes education class, and it was a huge eye-opener. They started talking about something called "portions." What is a portion, I wondered?

When I sat down to eat dinner previously, I had no sense of portions. If I had rice, I probably had two cups of rice. It was a big deal to weigh, measure, and more importantly, see what 4 ounces of meat actually looked like. What is a cup of something? To do this day, that is my main nutrition tactic. If I start to see my weight creeping up, I go back to measuring and weighing all foods again, and I regain my control.

The first time I weighed and measured everything out, I sat down with my plate in front of me. I looked down at my plate, and I realized something. My diabetes isn't going to kill me. As I looked at the portions on my plate, I realized; no, I was actually going to starve to death!

Truth to tell I wasn't full after eating it. But I was okay. Sort of. I was probably eating between 1500 and 1800 calories, so the portion was probably around 700 calories.

But at least now, I was aware and awareness is the key to change.

Basically, I thought the doctor and his health professional friends had thrown me a lifeline, a line that if I didn't grab onto I was surely going to drown.

Then, in addition to the nutritionist, I went to see a physical therapist. She said you're going to need to exercise. I laughed and said, "I'm 430 pounds, taking a shower is major exercise." She didn't buy that. "You need to start walking," she said seriously.

I had no choice. I had to get rid of the diabetes. At that point it had nothing to do with losing weight but everything to do with reversing the diabetes and escaping the needles.

So, I started to walk. I didn't go very far at first. To the end of the street and back, which in my case was about 100 feet! And even then I was out of breath. I did that every day, and soon I was walking around the block. I was shocked! Shocked about how quickly our bodies respond to activities like exercise when we do them every day. Within one month -- one month, at 430 pounds -- I was walking a mile. Yes, one mile!

That's insane! I thought it was incredible. I never looked back.

I walked every day; I tracked my food. For a while in the beginning, I did water aerobics, too. I kept this regimen up and my motivation by doing one other really critical thing.

I focused on taking my weight off 10% at a time.

When I was 430, that meant I had to lose 43 pounds. I knew I could do that. When that came off, I weighed 387 pounds, which meant I needed to lose 39 pounds. I can do that. Then I weighed 348, which meant I needed to lose 35 pounds. I can do that. Then I weighed 313, which meant I had to lose 32 pounds, which I did. Then I was 281.

And I did this in one continuous phase. I didn't lose 10% of my weight to a goal and then stop for a few weeks. The moment I reached a goal; I calculated my next goal, the next ten per cent, and was right back at it. No stopping. It was do-able.

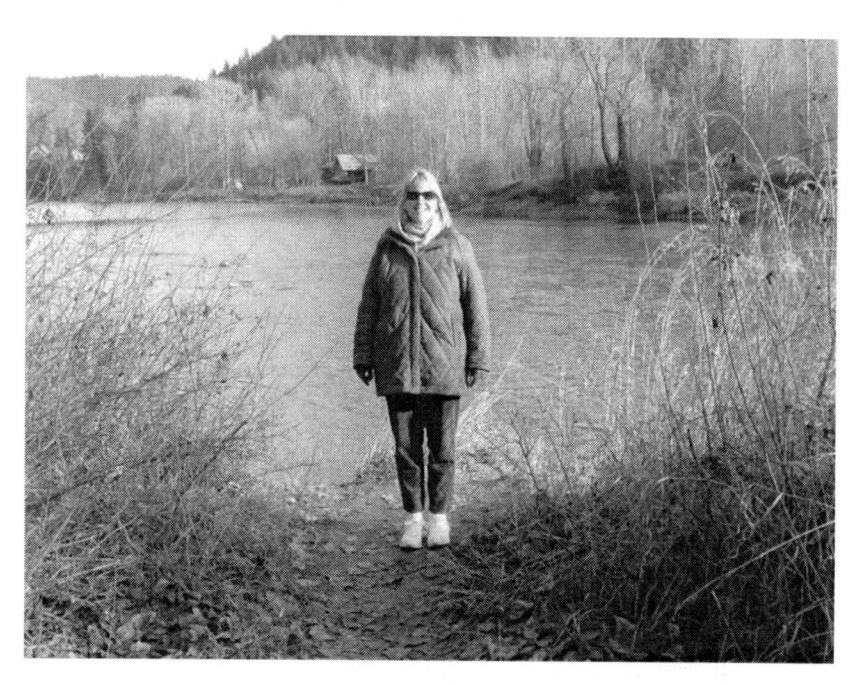

The more I lost, the more confident I was that I could lose more than the 10%. It didn't seem too long before I realized, "Wow, I could do this!"

It occurred to me that I could even be a "normal" weight. And all of that happened because the doctor didn't tell me I had to lose all my weight, or 200 pounds, or even 100 pounds. Just *some* of the weight.

So, in the end I lost 228.5 pounds. And I did it 10% at a time.

I lost my first 100 pounds in nine months. I lost my second 100 pounds in a year. The last 30 pounds took me another year. Just under three years in total.

When I watch the Biggest Loser, I sometimes marvel at how much weight the contestants lose. Then my husband reminds me that I lost even more, and I think, 'Oh yes, that's right; I did didn't I."

Some people lose 10 pounds at a time, but I had too much weight to lose. Moreover, the 10% was significant for me in terms of disease risk reduction. I was getting healthier with each 10%.

Interestingly, my health problems all virtually disappeared within the first 50 pounds, or about 10%. Today my cholesterol and blood pressure are perfect. I'm no longer diabetic. My numbers are great.
I actually started drawing down on my meds around the fifty-pound weight loss mark. The last medication they took me off was the Metformin for diabetes. In fact, the only reason my doctor kept me on it, as long as he did, is that it is meant to aid in weight loss. My doctor said, "You don't need this anymore but it's not going to hurt you to stay on it."

I didn't adjust my caloric intake when I exercised then, or now. I truly believe that I am addicted to food. If I start messing around with portions and calories, I'm asking for the addiction to fire up again. I have to keep it simple. I can't overthink it. That's a recipe for disaster. That's 300 calories turning into 900 calories.

Yes, I wish I had been addicted to alcohol or heroin, not food. There's no escape. Given the choice of a baked potato or a piece of pie, I'll choose the potato. But give me a choice between nothing and the pie, the pie will win. I definitely lean towards the bread and the carbs.

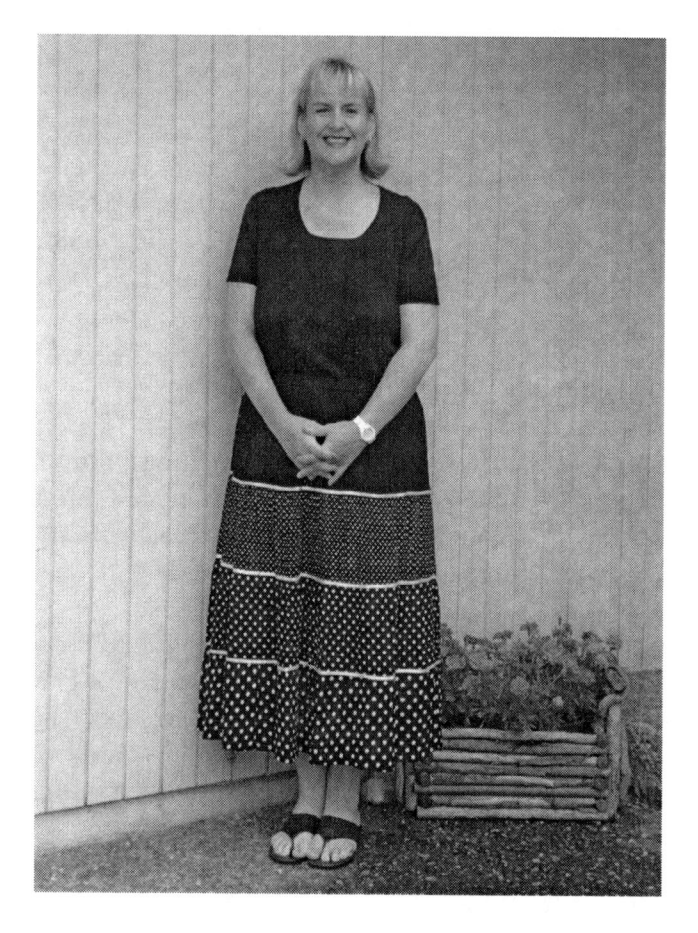

The nutritionist said, "I want you to eat your protein first, then your vegetables, then your fruit. If there's room left in the eating plan, then you can have carbs." Funny, I'd always eaten those food groups in the reverse order. I'd start with the starches and work my way back to the protein.

My husband's support was incredible. It was perhaps not so much about what he did do as what he didn't do. He never bothered me about my weight. He never questioned me or prompted me with "Are you sure you want to be eating that?" My husband never said anything. Not one word. We've been married 31 years and the only comment I can remember him making came after I had achieved my weight loss and became more active. Then, he commented how much fun it was now that I had energy and mobility, and we could do things together.

I did 90% of my exercise in the morning because I found that if I didn't get it in then, it probably wouldn't happen. I would get up, do my walk, get it over with and then get on with my day. Sometimes that didn't happen. And if on those occasions, I came home and said 'do you want to go for a walk or a bike ride?' my husband was more than willing to support me and come along.

"Sure, I'll go," he said. Always.

He is a facilitator even to this day. If I'm flagging in my resolve he will say, "Come on let's go for a walk." He never commented on weight. Not even, "You look skinny today," which in my mind would have meant I must have looked fat yesterday.

No, my husband is not a diplomat. I realize how hard it must be not to comment. I would find it difficult to be so quiet. For example, my brother has now gained weight, and I find it extremely hard not to comment or advise him. I'd love to say to my brother, "C'mon Randy, let's do this or don't do that," but I've learned to bite my lip. It's hard.

I walk about three miles every day. Some days I can do it in 45 minutes, other days it takes an hour. I've tried the gyms and the classes but for me and my schedule, I like to walk on my own, go at my own pace. I just like to walk out my door and go. No hassle. No driving to the gym. No socializing at the gym. Just out my door. It needs to be that easy otherwise I won't do it.

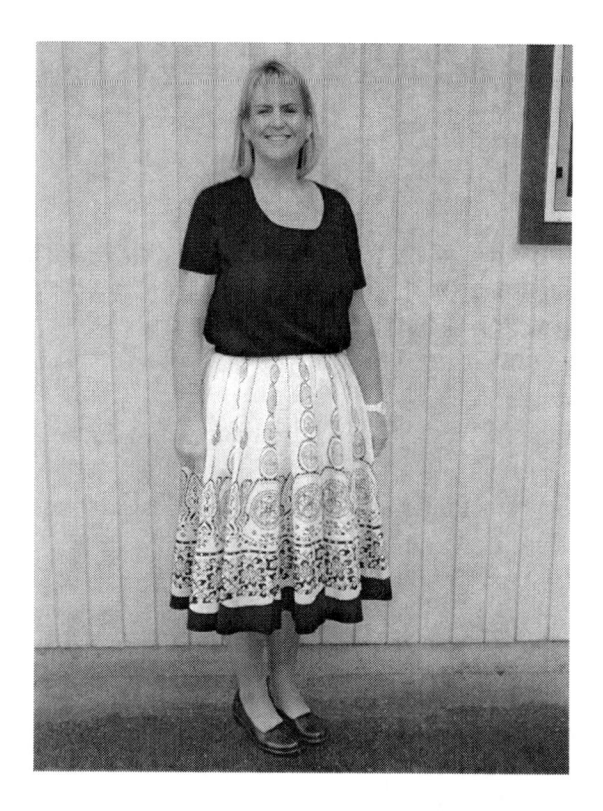

I did enjoy water aerobics but one thing that happened when I lost all my weight, was that my body temperature dropped, and I got cold. The water at the public pool where I did my water aerobics was also cold and I would just go in there and shiver. So I don't do that now, and I don't need to. I love walking. I have rain gear; I live in Oregon for goodness sakes. Rain doesn't stop me.

I reached my goal weight on December 30, 2010, which means I've maintained my loss for more than three years. The doctor's office is pretty amazed, not so much about losing the weight but keeping it off over a long period of time.

Not that losing was easy. During my weight loss, I reached a plateau and really freaked out. I went to see a psychologist, and I was truly stressing about the plateau. She asked me, "During your life, how many times have you maintained your weight loss?" I have never maintained weight loss. Well, she pointed out that's what's happening. "This isn't a plateau to be scared of; it's a maintenance phase to be proud of."

Wow!

These were the last 30 pounds, and I had been stuck for several months. But in an instant, this woman transformed my fear into a cause for celebration. I bawled. Right there and then I started to cry. It looked like she was used to it.

Then, soon after, the rest of the weight started to come off.

There's no question that maintaining it is harder than losing it. It's just tough finding that balance.

One huge factor was that I joined a wonderful support group -- TOPS. Support is a very important part of losing weight. We all need a pat on the back when we are doing well and encouragement when we're not. As overweight people, we tend to beat ourselves up anyway, so we need more than ever to be lifted up when down. TOPS members lifted me up. The unconditional and unbiased support is something I've never received before in a weight loss group or program. From the moment I walked into my first meeting, I felt like I belonged and that these people wanted me there. Every time I wanted or needed support, my TOPS members were there for me. They cried with me and laughed with me. They cheered me up and cheered me on.

The weekly weigh-ins were very important to keep me on track and accountable. Accountability is the key to weight loss. When I would think about eating something that wasn't the best for me, I would think again because I knew that I had to weigh in and be accountable for my actions. I also think it is the key to keeping the weight off. Facing the scale each and every week makes us face the facts.

TOPS also made losing weight fun. The contests and games, the charms and honors really boost your self-esteem and make you want to keep trying. TOPS members are really there for one another. I can't over estimate what TOPS means to me.

For me, it's all about my health. I don't want to be sixty and in a nursing home. I have fear, almost panic, about relapsing. I realize that motivation seems fickle. Some days are tough. But I have found a way to deal with them.

When my motivation is weakening I make a concerted effort to focus on my success. I look at pictures to remind myself of how far I have come. I talk to myself about my health, diabetes, and needles. It has gotten easier to do that with practice. I am grateful for this life -- walking, bike riding, energy, and I don't want to go back to the way I was before. I don't want to think about whether I'm going to break a chair or be able to walk around a city. I don't want my family to go back to that life, either. For better or worse, they have suffered, too. If they could have lost the weight for me, it would have been gone years ago.

Making my efforts about my health made a huge difference. When it was all about the scale, it didn't work. When it was about being healthy, the whole dynamic changed along with my success.

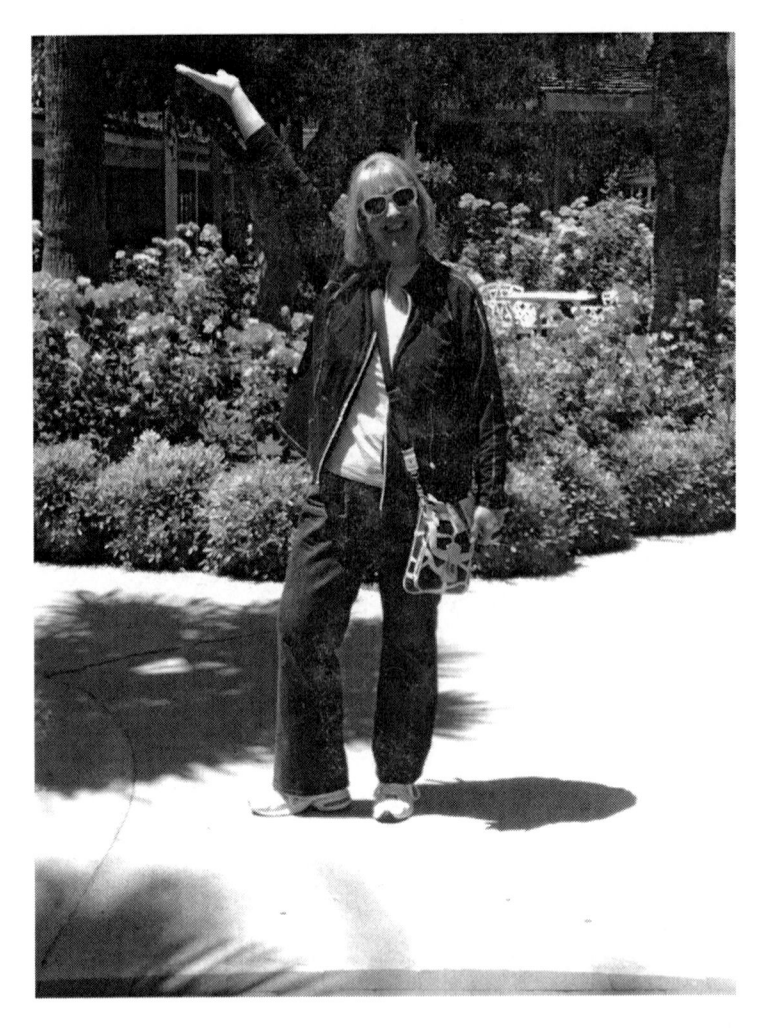

I still look at the number on the scale, but it's not the driver. If I've done the right thing, I don't freak out if the scale goes up. I weigh weekly. I used to get on and off the scale. If I lost weight, it was an excuse to eat more. If I gained weight, it was an excuse to eat more. If the scale stayed the same, it was an excuse to eat more. Every week, mom would ask me about my weight. I realized I can't do that. If I don't lose as much as she expects, I'll feel bad and mad. I can't do this. Please don't ask. I don't want to report. So, about half way through my final weight loss saga, she stopped asking. She actually quit asking me about my weight loss. Good, because it's not about the weight loss.

I'm still afraid of needles -- Thank God. I can't identify why, but even as a child I had this phobia. The idea of stabbing myself, once let alone multiple times a day, I simply can't wrap my head around that.

I still think of myself as exactly the same person. I think I look the same. I know logically I don't, but it seems that way. One of the biggest differences is my energy level. Recently, we went to San Diego and went kayaking. That's something I would never have dreamed about doing before. For one thing, I probably wouldn't fit in the boat.

Another benefit is that sometimes I run into people, and they don't know who I am. That's fun. It's good because there are some people I don't want to acknowledge, and I can walk right past them! Other times, it's fun to see the surprise on people's faces when it finally dawns on them who I am.

I don't feel any different. I was also sociable and had friends even at 430. I didn't have the luxury to isolate myself. I am still busy in church and at work, like before. But there's definitely way less stress and anxiety at this weight. I had lots of worries at 430. Will I fit in the seat? In the booth? What do people think?

Another plus; clothes shopping is now a blast. Previously, if I found one shirt that fit, I'd buy one of every color. And when losing weight pretty quickly, I spent a lot of time at thrift shops and goodwill because, I hoped, the clothes were going to be obsolete pretty quickly.

Apart from coming off medications and reversing my diabetes and hypertension, my feet shrunk. I was a size 10 now I am a size 9. I think I saved myself from back, knee or hip problems by addressing my weight when I did, when I was still just young enough to avoid the onset of major problems.

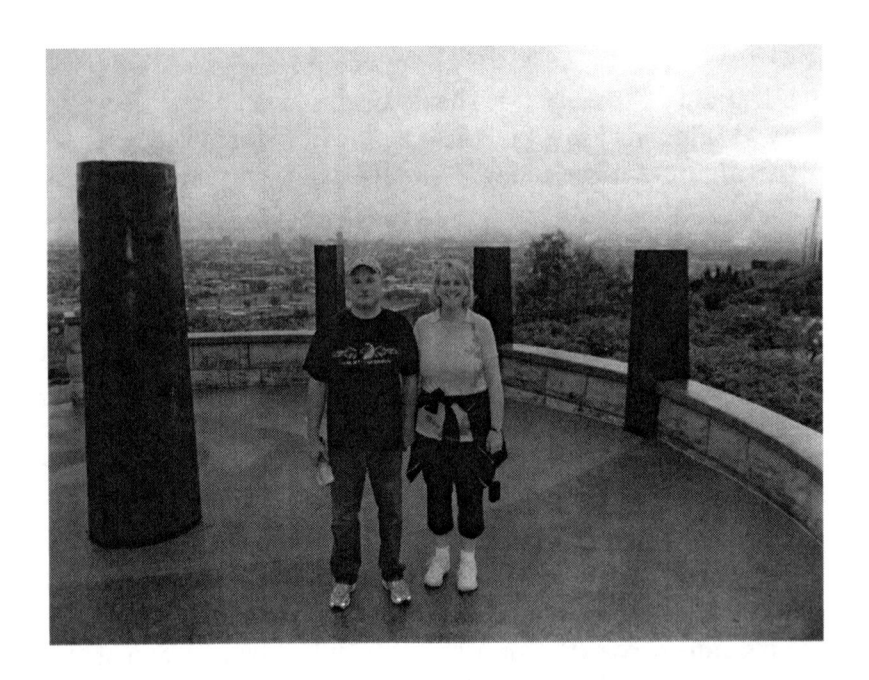

Another big physical benefit came when I had some excess skin removed. That removal of an apron of skin changed my life, almost more than weight, though, of course, if I hadn't lost the weight, I wouldn't have the need to remove excess skin. Yep, I had a big apron of skin that didn't go away. In fact, it got worse as I lost weight. Near my goal, my doctor said that the skin removal would lose 20 pounds, which just happened to be the amount I had to lose to reach my goal. I was ticked when I had the procedure in the fall of 2010, and the amount removed weighed just 15 pounds! But that procedure really changed my life. I could move, exercise, and wear shirts that didn't need to cover up extra skin. Most of all, it was the removal of embarrassment.

I might have lost the weight without TOPS; I don't know. But one thing I do know is that with TOPS, I will keep it off and my TOPS pals will be there for me through thick and thin.

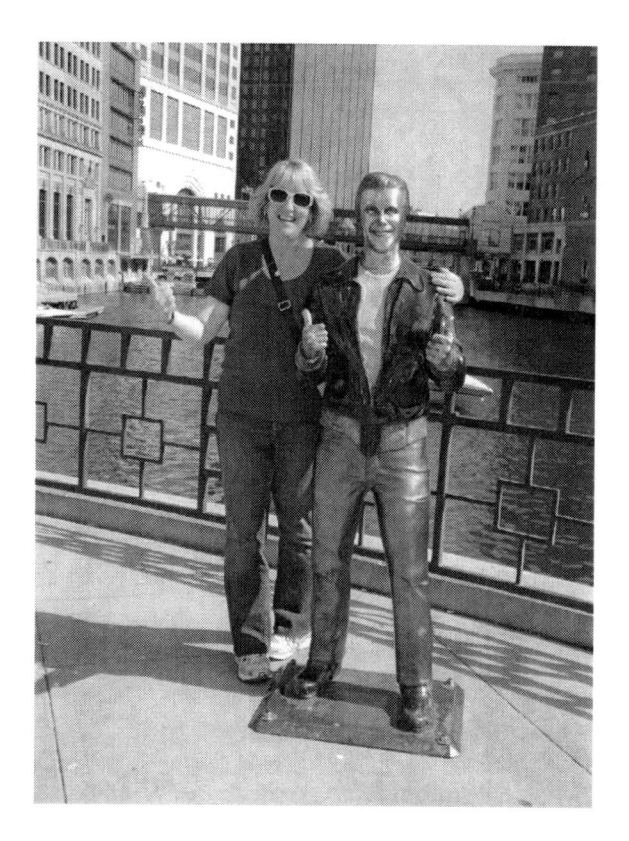

If I can lose that much weight, anyone can. Take it 10% of the time. Do it for your health. Find support. Get informed. Avoid denial. Be active. Remind yourself of your real motivation. Find the right doctor. And being afraid of needles helps, too.

Greg Altilio

Muscle Power

October 5, 2012. I'm waiting in the pre-op room of a New Jersey surgical center. It has taken me a long while -- too long -- to get here, but now I'm on the verge of realizing the decision I made a few months ago. As I am laying here, I think about all the concerns people have told me about the surgery.

"It's a dangerous procedure; you could die."

"What will you do with all that extra, hanging skin?"

"You don't need something so drastic."

"You can do it by just eating right."

"The operation is the equivalent to open-heart surgery."

I am distracted as the anesthesiologist enters the room. The doc goes over the procedure and then asks me a question.

"Are you really 425 pounds?"

That's one of my problems. Sure, everyone could see I was big, but they saw me as NFL lineman big, not Two Plane Seats big. That deceived everyone for a long while but most of all, me.

I was born into an Italian family. Enough said. Sure some of my family were on the heavy side but nothing out of the ordinary. A cousin, Danny, had the bypass procedure a decade before me and has done OK. Danny's been supportive.

"You're going to do a lot better than me," Danny said to me one day when we were comparing notes.

The reason for the confusion and the deceptiveness of my weight is exercise, or to be more specific, weights. I weighed 70 pounds in second grade but really started to bulk up by the time I got to high school. When I graduated from high school, I weighed 280, which for a guy who is just six feet tall is a lot. But by then, I became a power lifter. My big frame was mostly muscle. Or so it seemed.

In college, my weight fluctuated, but I kept up the exercise and the lifting. After college, I took a job that required a fair amount of physical activity, and my weight stabilized. But when a few years later, I was promoted into a less physical job; the weight started to increase, even though I was still lifting weights. About that time, I also moved to south Jersey from the northern part of the state and started to spend a lot of time in the car doing "windshield time."

I honestly wasn't paying attention to what was really happening. I figured that my weight and life were what they were meant to be. I was really in denial. I figured if I could exercise and lift weights the way I was, I must be okay. No one challenged me on this. My friends admired my muscular frame and thought I looked like a football player.

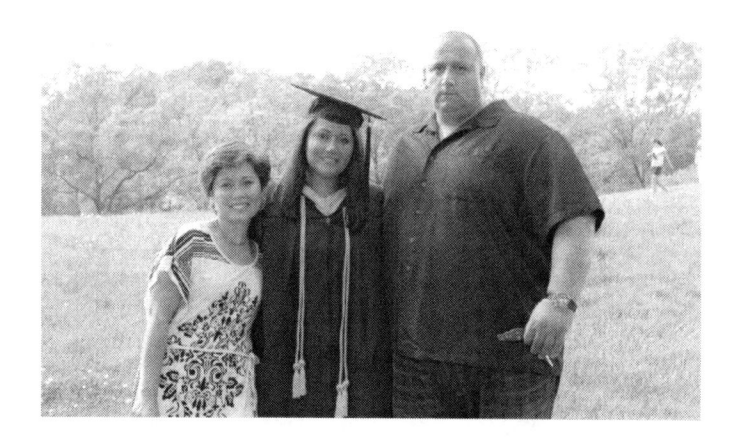

I always looked nice for work and did my job. On the surface, everything was okay, but that didn't tell the whole story. Beneath the surface, there was a different reality that I just didn't want to recognize.

When traveling by plane, I had to buy two seats. I was the guy you saw in the boarding line that you prayed wasn't sitting next to you. When I was in customer meetings, I looked for the chairs without arms, so I wouldn't be constrained, and could actually sit down. I actually panicked sometimes for fear there wouldn't be a seat that I could fit into. That's not what you ideally wanting to be thinking about going into a meeting.

When I went to the doctor's office and was weighed in, I covered my eyes and asked the nurse not to reveal the scale's truth. I became more isolated and wouldn't venture out much and certainly wouldn't go to the beach -- one of the prime advantages of having a home on the Jersey shore.

But there came a point when I couldn't turn a blind eye anymore.

My sleep deteriorated and I clearly had apnea. One day, I fell asleep at the wheel while driving to New England, and I ended up in a ditch. Boy, was I lucky! But even then my sleep apnea wasn't a wake-up call. There needed to be more.

My weight meant that I would sweat a lot, and I was really sensitive to that. I would often take three showers a day to compensate. The more I became aware of the perspiration, the more I sweated over it. I was also having trouble just bending over. That made tying my shoes literally a pain in the ass.

There was another reason shoes were a problem. I had edema in my legs, which swelled my feet badly. Even if I could bend over, my shoes wouldn't fit. My legs also swelled up big time, creating discomfort in my calf muscles and discoloring them, too. Sometimes they were almost black. My feet were often numb. My blood pressure shot up. It takes a lot to pump blood around a 450-pound body. I won't sugar-coat it; I was pre-diabetic, too.

You can avoid mirrors, but it's harder to ignore pain. I was getting the message loud and clear. I started to see my problems in other people. Frankly, it scared the hell out of me.

My job as a national account manager for a large, beverage company took me to casinos. Something strange started to happen there. I began noticing the older patrons at the casinos. In wheelchairs. With oxygen tanks. Without legs. Was I really willing to gamble that my physical problems weren't a gruesome sign of things to come? Was I going to end up like these guys? Sitting in a wheelchair barely able to play the slot machines?

My concern couldn't be contained any longer. My worry began to expand and crackle like popcorn in a microwave. It couldn't be ignored.

My father had died of cancer of the liver, largely because he spent a lifetime working around chemicals. Now, I began to think of the fat that surrounded my organs as toxic material, too. Doctors will tell you that is not an inaccurate assessment. A lot of fat around your organs makes them vulnerable. The more I saw fat as toxic, the more I knew had had to do something.

I came to realize that I wasn't living. More than that, I knew that if I didn't lose weight, I'd die. I felt as if my back was really against the wall. I knew I would have to do something, so I started to research obesity and obesity treatments.

My wife, Carmella, is 4"11 and about a quarter of my weight. I've eaten bigger sandwiches than she weighs. She has always been very supportive. So are my wonderful, college-age kids, Nicole and Anthony. They would do anything to help me, and now that meant helping me get help. They really encouraged me.

My son Anthony, 21, has always been active, athletic and healthy. He has always been vigilant about his well-being, exercising regularly and taking care of himself. He is a health science major at Quinnipiac College in Connecticut. One time when visiting him, I just couldn't make it up the dorm stairs to see his room. That hurt.

My daughter Nicole, 23, is pursuing a Master's degree in education. She, too, takes care of herself and is supportive of me in every way.

One of my aunts stepped up, too. She was very concerned about my weight. She actually referred me to a local weight loss and bariatric surgery group. I made an appointment.

At the clinic, I was introduced to a nutritionist. She was, quite frankly, amazed at how active I was. She told me that I probably could eat 4000 calories a day and not gain weight -- if I ate the right way.

But I wasn't eating the right way. I would eat some protein when I first awoke and after my workouts, but then I wouldn't eat until the end of a day, when I had a large, unhealthy meal.

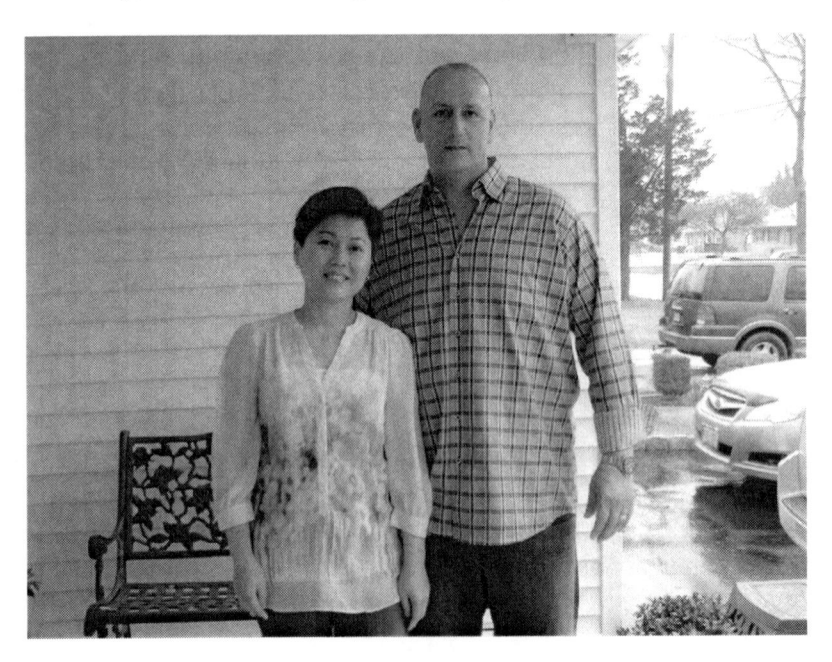

The nutritionist told me that the way I was eating was slowing down my metabolism. As a result, even though I was active, I wasn't losing the weight.

Armed with a food plan that required eating balanced meals several times a day, and a commitment to the weight-loss surgery, I lost 30 pounds in two months.

I learned that, typically, doctors doing bariatric surgery require potential patients to lose some weight prior to the surgery for two reasons. One, the less fat around the tissues and under the skin, the less complicated the surgery tends to be. Secondly, the medical team wants to be assured that the patient is willing to make the lifestyle changes that are necessary for weight loss. I discovered that weight-loss surgery effectively provides patients like me with a window in which to make changes. Surgeons will tell you that you have to cut out the bad habits because you can't make a habit of being cut.

There were those who questioned my decision, as mentioned in the beginning, but I was resolute. After listening to the doctors and doing the research, I opted for the gastric bypass surgery. The sleeve and the lap band didn't appeal to me, and the bypass has the best record of success. I was committed.

My wife, Carmella, unlike some of the other people I knew, was completely supportive. She tends to listen to, and trust, medical opinion. The kids were on board, too.

As I chatted with the anesthesiologist in the pre-op room that night in October, I was ready and comfortable. Mine was the last surgery of the day, and I hadn't eaten for more than twenty-four hours. I actually walked into the operating room. I remember joking with the doctor and the nurses, and then, nothing.

I got back into the post-op room at around 8pm.

"Get up as soon as you can," said the nurse.

At midnight, I was up and walking around. One small step for a man, one huge leap for me.

It wasn't long before I was back home and into my schedule. Within two weeks, I was back at the gym and into my morning routine. You may think it's brutal, but I enjoy it. I'm up at 3:30, at the gym by 4 (yes, believe it or not there are other fanatics in the gym at that time!) and out after two hours of a comprehensive workout that includes resistance and cardio exercises. Then, it's off to work after a protein-based breakfast.

It's a routine that I have kept up religiously. In fact, now eighteen months later, it has become even more structured. Along with a general, comprehensive work-out, which begins with thirty minutes on the elliptical, I target specific muscle groups each day.

Monday, it's biceps, Tuesday, the chest, Wednesday, triceps, Thursday, shoulders, Friday, back, Saturday, stomach, Sunday, legs.

I simply can't lie in bed. Once I'm awake, I need to get moving. Carmella thinks that I'm out of my mind, but I say, if you have a vice, this is a good one to have. Actually, I don't have many vices. I've never been a drinker, a smoker, or a drug user. Just a foodie.

With a reduced appetite and an increased commitment, I found the transition to regularly scheduled eating of healthy foods a piece of cake -- or rather a bowl of oatmeal. The foods I used to devour no longer interest me.

Previous staples, like macaroni and cheese and pizza, are no longer appealing. I can take them or leave them. And I choose to leave them. If I have a steak at all, it has to be accompanied by an entourage of vegetables.

I have also eliminated the bread and the so-called white foods -- pasta, confectionery -- that cause blood glucose to spike rapidly but fall just as fast, creating lethargy and a craving for more of the same.

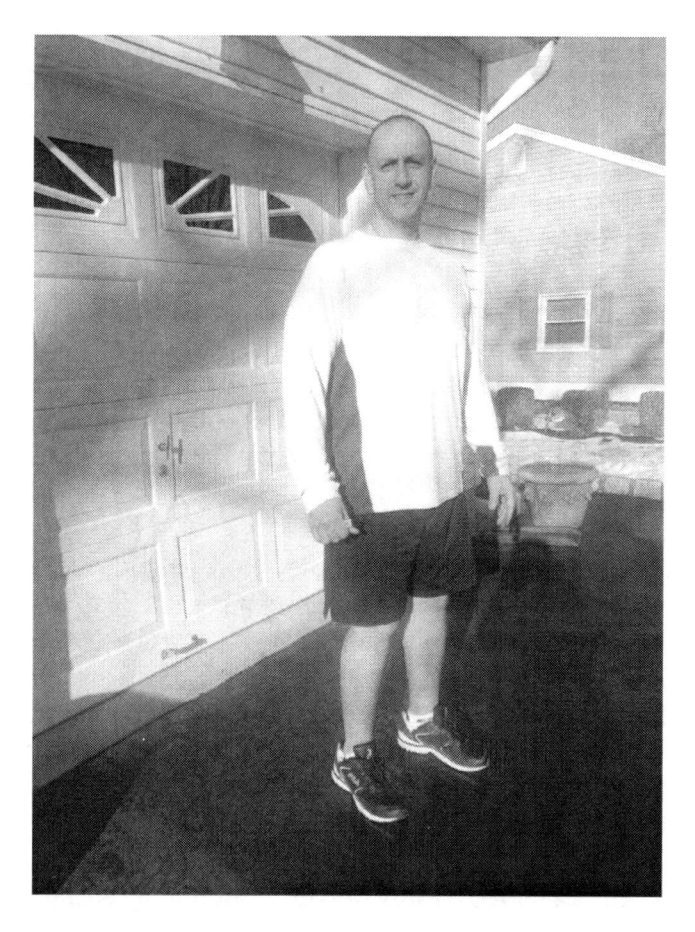

Oatmeal, fruit and nuts are my standard breakfast fare. Soup and vegetables are my common lunchtime meals. Yogurts, protein bars and drinks are the usual snacks. Dinner is varied, almost always with vegetables. Sashimi has become a favorite.

A month after the surgery, Hurricane Sandy struck the New Jersey coast, notably damaging the Point Pleasant area just a few miles from my home.

The whole area was without electricity for two weeks but there was no power outage at my house. We were thoughtful enough to buy a generator. I had the energy to keep my routine going. And energy is a big issue.

I'm on my feet all day, at the gym for two hours, but I never get tired now. Previously, low energy was a huge problem. That is no longer an issue.

Once on my exercise regime and regular, healthier eating, the weight started to roll off. A lot of it.

I've lost 185 pounds in eighteen months to be exact.

Yep, at first I didn't notice any changes even though I was down thirty or forty pounds. Then it reached a point when I didn't quite believe the person looking back at me from the mirror was really me. Sometimes, I'm shocked.

So, there's no more hiding out, no more avoidance, no more isolation. That all took an awful lot of energy, and deep down, I was unsettled if not downright miserable.

In the summer, I work outside in the yard, without a shirt. I'll walk the beach. My wardrobe has greater variety. I am much more comfortable driving, mentally and physically -- and I drive 60,000 miles a year. I only need one plane seat.

Apart from my commute, I also travel more. On a recent trip to the Philippines to visit with my wife's family, I got a pass to my brother-in-law's gym and was able to keep up my workout routine. Where no such facilities exist, I adapt. For example, on a recent trip to California, I made the best use I could out of the equipment available in the hotel fitness room.

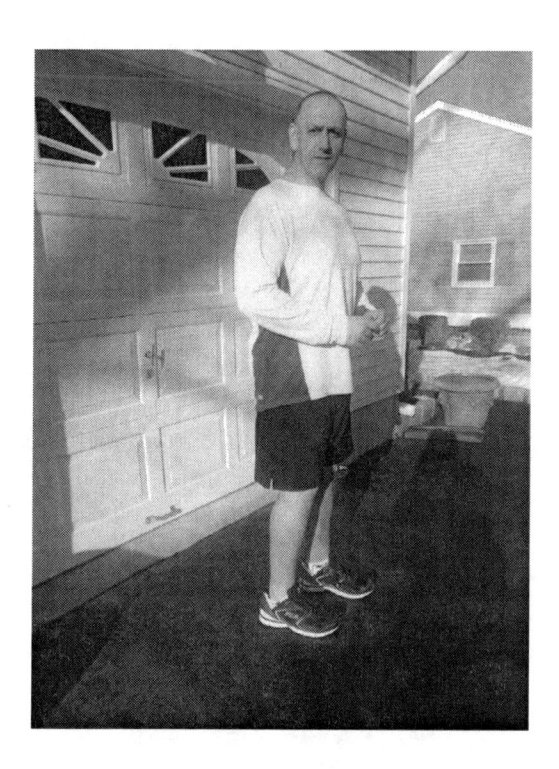

I am always on. I've learned that you have to be. I can't wing it. I need to stay with my routine.

If you have had a lifelong weight problem, I would definitely recommend the surgical procedure. The technology is available, so take advantage of it.

If you are obese, it's not *if* but *when* you will get ill. Do it, and do it as soon as you can. The younger you are, the better.

In many ways, I was an ideal candidate for the surgery. I had a strong workout ethic in place and was as fit as someone at my weight could be. That not only prepared me for the surgery but made my post-surgery lifestyle change that much easier. On a recent medical visit, my doctor said, "Greg, you're doing everything right." He added, "And don't lose any more weight."

I have also gotten a lot of support along the way. I had a supervisor at work, who was into fitness and was very supportive, even after he moved on to another company. And my customers, of course, notice the difference and are complimentary. My family have been there every step of the 'weigh'.

They see me differently.

I see myself differently, too.

I am much more comfortable in my skin.

My confidence has soared, and the self-doubt has melted away along with my adipose tissue. Not that fear doesn't lurk in the shadows, but in a funny way it helps.

Quite simply, I'm terrified of going back.

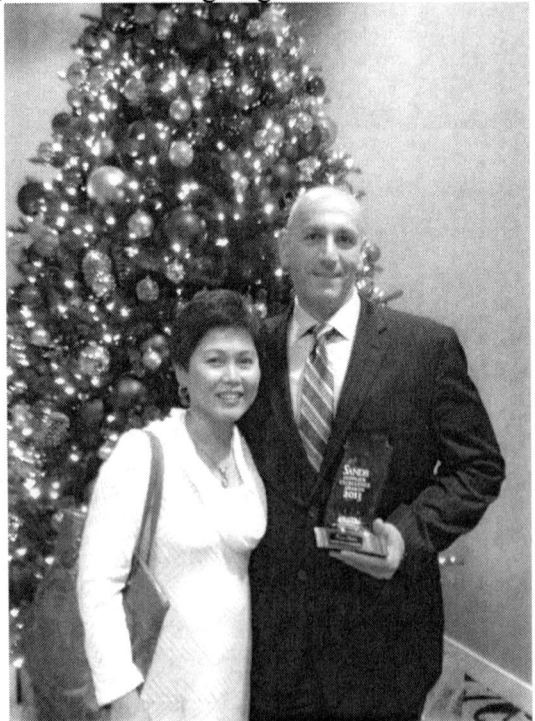

I've got a life now. And I'm not giving it up.

Susan Ames

The Power of Support

I was raised in La Mesa, near San Diego. There were a lot of females in the house. Apart from my mom, I had three other sisters, ranging from about eight years older to four years younger than me. With five women in the house, there was a lot of talk about weight.

My older sister Amy, younger sister, Tracy, myself, and my mom struggled with our weight, but we grew up pretty healthily. The house rule was that we couldn't have added sugar. It was sugar-free snacks and water rather than soda. I think this was mainly due to the fact that my parents didn't want four girls running around crazy, hyped up on sugar. We were always playing outside in our huge backyard and often walked down the street to the nearby elementary school to play kickball. However, there wasn't any real emphasis on exercise or even healthier nutrition apart from the sugar issue.

Weight was always a big subject. By the time I was 12 my weight had been up as high as 166, and at the time I was only about five feet tall. There was a lot of stress at home that eventually led up to my parents' divorce. It was a struggle, and I was out of control. My mom was worried about me. She and a great aunt were going to TOPS, Take Off Pounds Sensibly; a local weight loss support group. So, at the end of middle school, during my rising high school freshman summer, I went along, too.

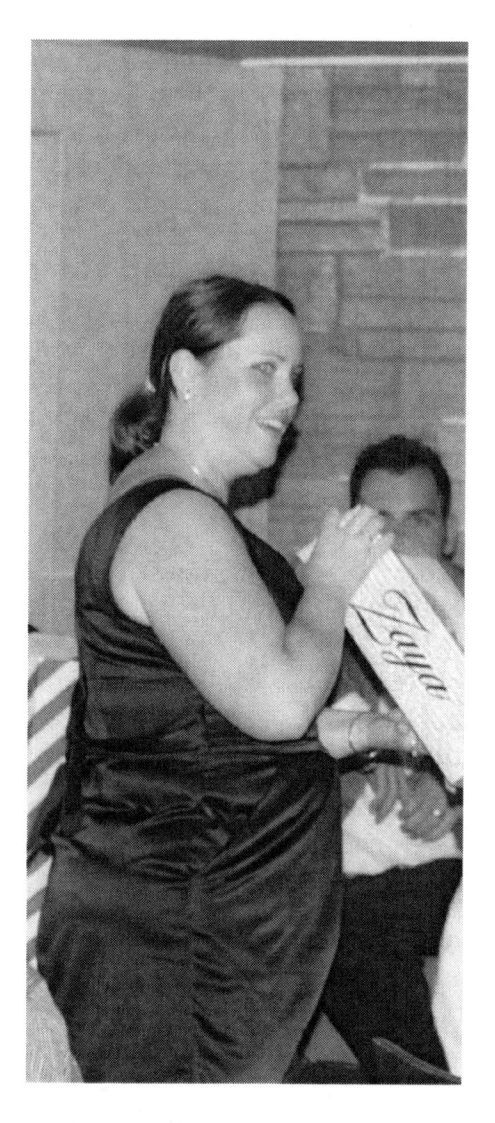

TOPS is an international weight loss support group with thousands of chapters, mostly in the US and Canada. The groups are inspiring and empowering and the one I went to was no different. The group was comprised of almost all women, and most of them were old enough to be at least an aunt if not another grandmother. But they were incredibly supportive! I think they were thrilled to have a teenager in the group, and I felt a lot of love from all of them. With their encouragement, inspiration, sensible advice about portions, and time spent playing softball, walking and exercising to video tapes; I dropped thirty pounds. Back at that time, TOPS had Area Recognition Days (ARD) as well as State Recognition Days (SRD). I actually won first prize at ARD in the teen division with 37.5 pounds lost in one year, and I won second place in the state. My mom also did well during this time and got into the best shape that I can remember.

I was extremely shy at this age and only had two or three friends while in middle school. Not only did I have a weight problem I had bad acne, too, which didn't help. I was short, round, and shy. I was self-conscious, and the teasing didn't help. I did do well in school, but that didn't make things any better for me socially. If anything, it made it worse.

Having dropped the excess weight; however, I started high school with a bit more confidence. I even tried out for the softball team and made some new friends. My freshman year was good, a big improvement over the previous year. I was emerging a little from my shell but was still one of the shier kids. Sophomore year was very similar, and I even met a boy and we started to date. Junior year, however, was very different.

I became pregnant.

The school actually wanted me to leave and get my education elsewhere. I guess they thought I was a bad advertisement. However, my mom had just got divorced and there wasn't any money for me to go somewhere else, so despite the school's opposition; I stayed.

Despite the school's outlook, I didn't feel like an outcast. I wasn't looked down upon. The girls in my class and in the school thought it was exciting and cool -- I'm not sure why, but they did. They watched my body grow, and they probably got a good education in pregnancy.

I did put on about fifty pounds during my pregnancy. I got good care from my doctors, and they thought I was in great shape. They said that I was the healthiest teen they had ever seen. I kept exercising through my pregnancy, although there were times when I capitulated to the inevitability of the weight gain and rationalized away excessive consumption as the result of having to eat for two. But I was keeping a food journal, monitoring my portions and walking a lot.

I eventually had my daughter, Katie, during my junior year and finished my schooling from home. In fact, I needed only to take electives and completed all my work by March of my senior year.

Being a single mom at such an early age was challenging. But I had my three sisters and my mom to help. It was the village concept; one of them took over when I needed to work.

My boyfriend and I were committed to get married, but neither of our parents wanted us to do that until we had graduated from high school. So we were actually married the day after our Senior Prom! Needless to say we didn't go to the prom. We had more important things to do the following day. For a while, we lived with my in-laws before we could afford a small place of our own. I got a job working at Long's drugstore.

The people at Long's were just as interested in my experience as a young single, mom as my high school friends. They were also as supportive as my TOPS group.

I lost a lot, but not all, of my pregnancy weight, and I was feeling pretty good. I even enrolled at community college and started my work towards an accounting degree. Then my husband decided that he wanted to join the Marine Corps Reserves and went off to boot camp. That was a big change. Although I had a lot of support, this was the first time I had lived alone, just me and Katie. It made me think.

When my husband returned from his basic training, it was obvious to both of us that we had married far too young, and it really wasn't going to work out. We separated and I went to live with Amy, my oldest sister, for a while until I could afford a small apartment, which I was able to do within a few months. So here I was, a single mom, working retail part-time and going to school to get some accounting qualifications.

One day, I was in my accounting class and complaining about working in retail. There was a girl in my class who was already working in finance and was back in school just to brush up on a couple of topics. She was working in her mom's construction business, and before long she had connected me with one of the subcontractors, and I was soon getting paid to help out with bookkeeping. This was great experience as I was learning first-hand the practical aspects of the accounting business while still in college. It also got me out of retail and onto a professional path. This was in the nineties where businesses were going digital with their spreadsheets but still partly stuck in old accounting habits. So I got double experience in keeping the old-style general ledger while also learning new computerized programs like Quattro Pro. Unfortunately, my employer at the time wasn't into Microsoft, so I had to adapt later.

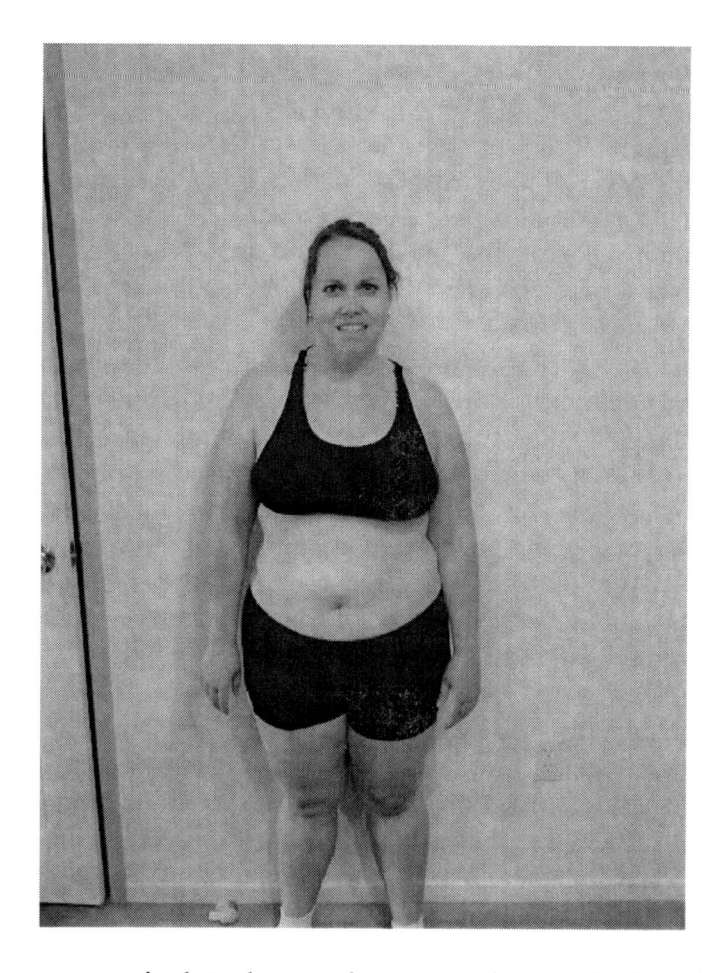

I was very excited to be on the accounting track. Initially, my weight was good. I didn't have much of a social life for a number of reasons. I was still pretty shy. I was a very busy single mom. I was still going to school. More importantly, perhaps, I had decided after the break-up of my marriage that I wasn't interested in re-marrying. I had decided that it would just be me and Katie, and I would become dedicated and be the best mom and person I could be. I had the support of my sisters, my mom and the people in my complex were helpful, too. They knew I was a single mom and helped out in different small ways, like taking my groceries up the stairs to my apartment and generally making sure we were safe.

I was busy and as a result my exercise began to fall by the wayside. I simply had too many other priorities. I was inconsistent with my food, too. During these years, my weight typically vacillated between and 150 and 210. I topped out at 215.

I had a couple of different accounting jobs but landed a more permanent position at a real estate company. In 2006, I finally got my accounting degree and for the first time since Katie was born, I actually had some free time. What would I do with it?

My sister Lisa's idea was to run a marathon! She knew some people who were preparing for one, in part to raise money for charity. We went to an event about the marathon and sponsorship with not much intention of doing either, but then we hadn't seen the promotional video. When we saw an eight-year-old girl with a shaved head saying she was going to do everything in her power to beat her cancer, we were hooked. The girl wasn't much younger than Katie. So we signed up to be a sponsor and run the marathon. Neither of us had run before. Not even a mile.

Marathon training was amazing. It brought my sister and me so much closer together. We were up at six in the morning, running together, sharing stories of her travels and my motherhood. Up to that point in her life, she hadn't been interested in having children but that time together, along with her husband's encouragement, changed her views about it.

The Team in Training organization was fantastic, teaching us and other non-runners how to be runners, or even run-walkers. We started slowly, of course. When we were told that in a few weeks we were going to run eight miles, we were daunted, if not cynical. But when that time came, we were ready, prepared by weeks of increasing distances, and literally took the eight miles in our stride.

The time with my sister, the increased levels of fitness, new friends, and a sense of accomplishment, all made this an incredible journey. Then it was time for the race, which was officially the San Diego Rock 'N Roll Marathon. Despite the workouts, my weight didn't drop below 180.

The race started from downtown and six of us started out together as a group. Now, this wasn't the Olympics. We were singing songs, telling stories, discussing what we were going to eat when we finished. We even stopped along the way to have photos taken with friends and supporters. My mom and sister followed along, easily distinguishable by the banner they had made. Katie was there, too, proud of her mom and aunt but not too interested in following in their footsteps.

As the race ground on, we were getting exhausted. We were the real endurance runners. The leaders were only running for about two hours, but we were out there for nearly six! We supported, cajoled and helped each other and all crossed the finish line together.

Running a marathon will change your life. You can't go back to being a non-runner after that. I have done several more since then. Crossing the line was very special and gave me an amazing sense of accomplishment. Of course, my friends and family were excited, too. And there was someone else to help me at the finish line.

We had been doing intensive training and our longest runs on Saturday mornings, which meant there was no partying or social activity on Friday evenings. About a month before the race, however, our Saturday schedule was moved to Sunday. At last, a chance to have some fun on a Friday night! In all honestly, I was still very definitely in my "I'm never getting married again" mindset but a friend of mine was having a birthday celebration, so a few of us met at a downtown bar.

Before long, a couple of guys came by and asked me to play some pool. They were both older guys, and they couldn't stop boasting about their important jobs. One of them was going on and on about his role at Qualcomm. They were pretty boring, and I was looking for a polite way to exit. As I did so, I saw a guy across the room, who was much more my age and my type. Our eyes made contact and before long I was sitting next to him making small talk.

We were getting along well, until my sister came and sat on my lap saying, "What are you doing with my girl-friend?" But Robert was too smart for that.

"You two look too much alike. I bet you're sisters."

I liked Robert, and I told him I could hang with him, but I had a very busy schedule, and he wouldn't be a high priority. He stuck around, and he was at the marathon finish line. He helped me off with my smelly shoes and sweaty socks -- then promptly did the same for my sister. Wow! Perhaps I need to reconsider this marriage thing? My Bachelor's degree graduation was around this time, too, and he came and met all my family at the same time.

I had been fine being on my own for almost ten years. In retrospect, I am glad that I took that time for myself and Katie, and that I didn't just jump back into the dating scene. Robert and I continued to date and after several months, it became clear to us that this was a serious and special relationship. Eventually, we moved in together while saving up for our wedding. I kept my running going and did a couple of half-marathons and ultimately three Rock 'N Roll marathons in a row. My weight was fairly stable, ranging from between 160 at my lowest and 180 at my highest.

Then my stability was shaken by another event that rocked my world. I had been working for the real estate company for eight years. After the slowdown in the economy, there had been a wage freeze, but I was getting frustrated and felt I deserved more money. My boss agreed and together we created a proposal for a salary increase. A short while later I was called into her office and was fully expecting to hear good news.

Instead, she told me the company was letting me go. I was in total shock.

The loss of income and the fact that the landlord wanted us out of his place, so he could renovate it, led to Robert, Katie and I, moving back into my family home to live with my mother. It was big enough and made a great temporary refuge. This also helped us with our wedding savings! But I was definitely unsettled, and my eating became erratic and the weight started to pile on. I eventually got a new job at a software company but trying to learn the ropes and make a good impression didn't help my stress or my eating.

My work for the software company involved a variety of start-up ventures. One of these was Healthy Circles, which enabled subscribers to keep all their medical information in one place, allowing easy access for physicians and even family members, as well as the ability to track medical progress, like blood-sugar. I, however, wasn't making much medical progress.

Robert and I married in March of 2012, a year before the company I worked for was acquired by Qualcomm.

Qualcomm is all about work/life balance. They have great corporate gym facilities, a terrific team of fitness professionals and a range of physical activities available before and after work hours. When I started at Qualcomm, I was back up to my heaviest, but it wasn't long before I took advantage of these great facilities.

I met with a personal trainer. We didn't just work-out and focus on fitness; we reviewed my nutrition, too. Soon, I was being mindful of my portions, checking my weight weekly at my local TOPS group, and training for another half marathon. But this time I had a secret weapon.

My husband has always been incredibly supportive of me. When I was laid off from the real estate company and was feeling stressed and depressed, he sat me down and told me that I actually could do a lot better, I had much more potential, and that I would eventually find a more satisfying and more rewarding position. That made me feel more cheerful and as it turned out, he was right.

Now, that I was more settled and ready to tackle my weight again, he offered to help in many ways.

First, he loves cooking and was ready to take over that role. He ensured we ate healthily, with clean foods in good portions.

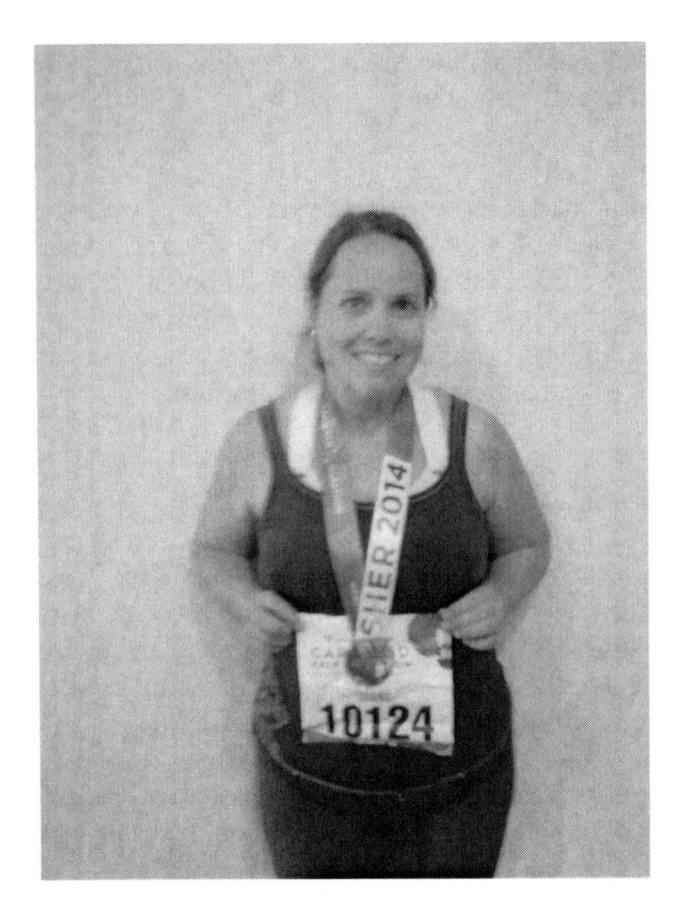

Second, he offered to remind me of my goals if he saw that I was straying from my committed path. It was really crucial that we discussed this in detail and came to an agreement about it. Robert really didn't want to be the food police; he wanted to help me realize my goals.

Some of my friends and family witnessed him commenting about my food choices, and they thought he was very controlling. When I told them we had an agreement, and that he was reminding me about my goals with my blessing, they completely changed their view. There's no question that had we not discussed and agreed on his approach; his comments would have been very irritating and counter-productive. I also knew he was coming from a place of love, not judgment. He wasn't saying, "don't eat that because you'll get fat and then I won't love you," he was saying, "you asked me to remind you not to eat that and I'm telling you because I love you."

Robert learned how to be a supportive partner watching his mother lose fifty pounds and completely change her lifestyle with the incredible support of her husband. They actually did that together and Robert and I did it together, too.

We read articles and books about nutrition together, and he adapted his cooking accordingly. Together, we learned more about portion sizes and eating clean. It was a complete team effort. He wasn't dictating to me; he was participating with me.

Since August of 2013, when we started our program, we have settled on a fairly limited diet of fish, chicken and occasionally some turkey with salad, fruits and veggies. Having a limited number of meal variations actually makes it easier physically and mentally. For one thing, our bodies are used to the food we're eating; we're not introducing any nutrition that is drastically different. And mentally we're not spending a lot of time wondering what to have, imagining different foods, and being tempted by our imaginations.

One thing that was difficult for me at first was dessert. Resisting desserts is super hard for me. Our solution? We decided to allow ourselves a 100-calorie dessert every evening. That could be some jello or a little pudding, just a taste of something. That has worked really well for me. I'm still getting healthy treats, but I am not feeling deprived. My usual goal is between 1200 and 1300 calories a day, increasing to 1600 calories a day when I exercise.

Robert also supported me with my exercise training goals and workouts. He made sure I stuck with my schedule. If I wanted to sleep in when I was meant to be at the gym, he would tell me that I needed to go to the gym. "Don't lose your momentum," he would say, lovingly.

The combination of the easy availability of great facilities and Robert's support has me as focused as I have ever been about my weight, fitness and overall health.

I lost weight every week over 24 weeks starting in August 2013. Yes, I lost weight over Thanksgiving, at Christmas and New Year! Constant support has made the real difference. It is so easy to lapse if left to oneself. It's easy to justify slacking off for any number of reasons. It so much easier doing it as a team. When there's a team, there's accountability. As I look back on my weight-loss efforts, I do really well when I have accountability. I did well as a teenager as a member of TOPS when I had all those 'aunts' supporting me.

Not only do I have Robert's support, people I exercise with at work also hold me accountable. They'll text me to tell me they are on the way to the gym, or to ask where I am, or ask me to join them. I also have returned to my local TOPS group to add even more layers of accountability.

So, on Mondays, and Wednesdays I do a forty-five-minute circuit at my work's gym, Tuesdays, I do weights and cardio for a ninety minute workout. Thursday is my TOPS weigh-in and meeting. Saturdays I also do Zumba and Body Pump, and I also do training runs, sometimes up to 11 miles, at the weekends.

I have lost almost fifty pounds in eight months and can really see a difference in my body. My body fat has fallen by 20%, and my muscle mass has increased by 20%. My resting metabolic rate has gone up to 1400 calories a day.

The wellness culture at work has made a huge difference. It has enabled me to take my fitness level way beyond what I thought was possible. The ease of access, the availability of the trainers, the small groups, the accountability, and the convenience of after-hours workouts, have all contributed.

Robert's love and support have been crucial. I can't imagine how someone could really lose weight if they had a spouse who was bringing junk food into the house, or were simply not interested, let alone unsupportive.

For Robert, it wasn't about my weight; it was about my self-confidence and self-esteem. I am so much happier with myself. I am no longer, short, round and shy. To emphasize how much of a team effort it had been, Robert himself has dropped 26 pounds since we started our program together.

There's been one other source of support that has made the world of difference to me.

Katie has paralleled Robert's support, She, too, has encouraged me and congratulated me, pushed me and inspired me. I know she is proud of me. I hope that as she makes her way off to college, she has learned the amazing power of family and group support.

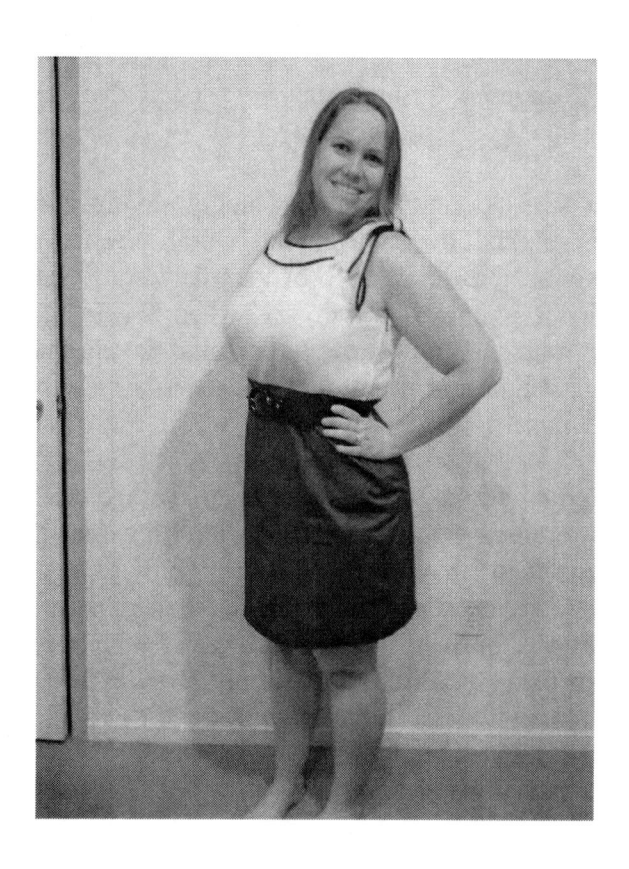

Thom Pulliam

A Vision Realized

I grew up in my early years in Arizona but moved to a suburb of Atlanta after fifth grade. Suburbia. I was there through high school and in 2007, I went to the University of Georgia and graduated from the journalism school in 2011. Since then, I have been working at a series of locations, working as a brand strategist.

After college, I was recruited to the Richards Group and lived in Dallas for three months. Then I moved to Santa Monica, near the beach for 18 months through July of 2013, then I was off to Manhattan, where I currently live and work.

Each of these stops along the way has taught me much about myself, the enormous role that the environment -- both physical and social -- plays in behavior and the science of manifestation. I have achieved the vision that I imagined for myself when I was 16 -- lifestyle, career track, friends, and most of all, personal development. And my health habits, weight and fitness have all been a huge part of how I have defined myself.

I can never remember being skinny or even average weight. I was an obese child. According to my Mom, I didn't have an appetite until first grade, and then I ballooned. In fourth grade, I wasn't bullied or mistreated, but my size was much bigger than most of my peers. I was living in a suburb of Phoenix. I wasn't athletic, did as little physical exertion as possible, and simply wouldn't do any activity that involved taxing my cardiovascular system. I was allergic to PE.

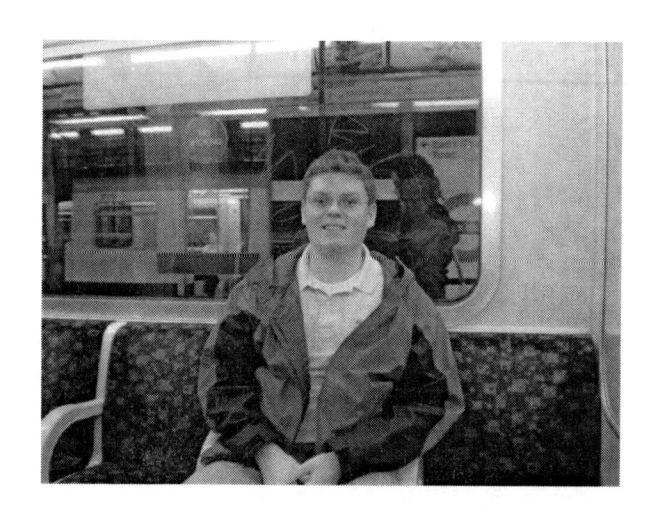

Phys. Ed. classes made me feel like a failure. I've always excelled at pretty much everything except P.E. You might remember the ropes climbing you had to do in PE? There were long ropes hanging from the ceiling, and you were meant to climb up them and flip over and climb down. I was never sure of the purpose of this exercise, and I still don't get it today. Moreover, nobody ever gave any instruction on how to do it. I could never do it. I hated it. I always tried to get lost at the back of the line, or somehow make myself invisible. I just didn't get it. And I was heavy to boot.

So I was shy of PE and in PE. I did a few team sports. When I was about six, I was in little league, but only for one season. It wasn't fun for me.

I continued gaining weight after we moved to Atlanta. There's a family history of obesity. My mother's whole side of the family is obese, and the assumption is that it is genetic. Or at least, that's what I thought until fairly recently.

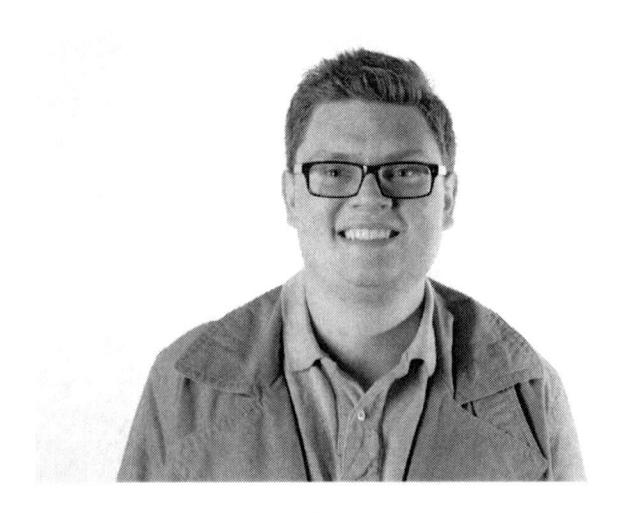

Not only have I now lost the weight I actually have had my DNA decoded through '23 and Me.' I was doing an assignment at work and to gather information on the company we were about to pitch; I tried out their genetic services. Their report of findings, which includes information about ancestral history, possible genetic mutations, and disease susceptibilities, was incredibly helpful to me. Their analysis showed that my genetic risk for obesity is right at the average, suggesting that I have no strong genetic predisposition for the condition. So, I believe that in my case, being obese had much more to do with lifestyle and environment. Knowing my genetic predispositions, has taken away the often easy excuse of being victim to my genes making me fat, which is what I had been led to believe prior, given my mother's family history.

The information was also empowering in that it showed me that I had no genetic impediments to losing weight or being healthy. If I put my mind to it and made the commitment, there was no reason at all why I wouldn't be successful. I would encourage anyone who struggles with their weight to do this testing. It's inexpensive, about $100, and the information is, in my view, invaluable.

By the time I was in seventh grade I weighed about 200 pounds. I was not happy. I avoided other kids and spent an awful lot of my time on my own, mostly playing video games in my bedroom. I had a whole setup in my room; a computer, a PlayStation, and a large

TV. My parents didn't force me to exercise or participate in physical sport. In any event, they had their own issues to work through, and I wasn't their priority. I was left to my own devices, literally and metaphorically. I was comfortable, but un-well.

The food at home was a typical All-American, suburban working-class junk diet. I remember when I was very young, sneaking into the pantry and taking chocolate ice cream bars and cokes. There was a lot of junk food around. I would sneak into the bathroom with Oreos, eat five or six at a time, and feel totally guilty about it.

My mom has been on various diets but has never been very successful, or maintained her weight loss for very long. When I was in the seventh grade, we teamed up and went to Weight Watchers together. Over the course of eight months, she lost 30 pounds, and I lost 50 pounds. This was a great success for us both. I was the youngest person in the meetings, which we attended each week according to the program. I learned better nutrition, got support and having my mom doing it with me was a great help as she was buying and preparing foods. We were learning and changing our behavior together. I started to go to the gym, too, and later would join the high school tennis team.

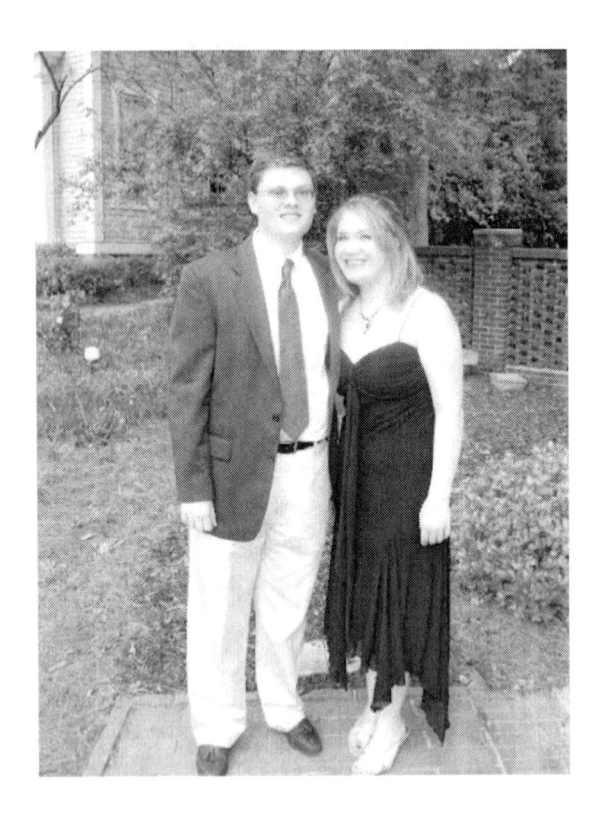

I got down to about 150 pounds as I was entering high school. It was the first time I ever remembered being at a normal BMI. This average weight also helped me be a little more sociable, but I still had a computer, PlayStation and other electronic gadgets in my bedroom, and they were a big distraction and an easy refuge. Moreover, Georgia is hot and the weather didn't encourage me to be outside. The culture is also one of driving everywhere, with less emphasis on physical activity outside, and more emphasis on watching sports and eating junk food. It's a culture of obesity, and it is accepted.

The lure of my electronic bedroom and the lack of activity conspired to increase my weight. By the end of high school, I had regained 30 pounds and was up to 180, not terrible, but not where I wanted to be.

When I was able to drive, I joined a gym. I got my first job at Publix supermarkets, too, at that time. Because I had generally been far less active than my peers, I wanted to increase my strength and tone up and that was the biggest allure of the gym.

I maintained my weight for six months, and on graduation, I was 6'0" and weighed 180. I moved to Athens, Georgia, when I started at the University of Georgia. I was in the dorm during my first year. The lifestyle was super unhealthy. In comparison to my peers, I was eating better and aligned to what I had learned in Weight Watchers – lots of veggies and no desserts, but there was still the all-you-can-eat meal plan. I was also surrounded by peers, who were eating junk food and drinking heavily, many times a week, sometimes binge drinking. I was eating a lot of calories, unhealthy calories, and not doing much exercise. When I left college, I weighed 250 and had grown to 6'2".

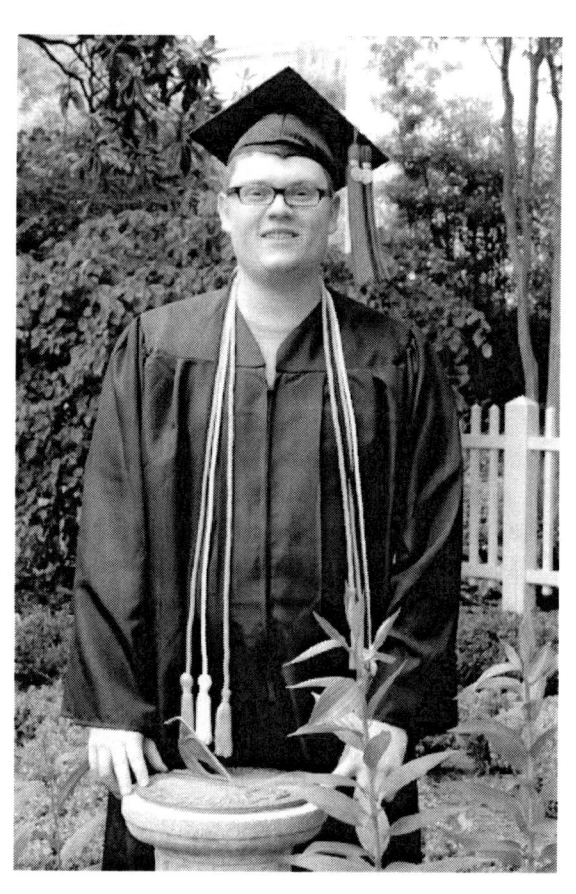

Through all this, I didn't have much confidence in myself as a mate and a partner. My energies were always thrown into my studies, my career and other activities. I didn't think I could be successful in a relationship or that anyone was attracted to me. I didn't isolate myself, but I didn't get much interest from others. I was active in my fraternity, Phi Kappa Theta, all four years, where I was on the executive board and was the House Manager. I was also a leader in the University Advertising Club, University advertising agency, and the University newspaper, so I was very active socially. I graduated in May 2011.

I went into marketing immediately. I had set myself up very well, with a good network and credentials that stood apart from my peers. I felt the biggest limitation I had to success was my weight, mostly for vanity reasons. I was 22, and I didn't want to be fat. I wanted to enjoy the life that vibrant cities could offer and attract others. Moreover, the ad industry is very image driven, and I didn't think it would help my career to be seen as unhealthy. I needed to look the part I wanted to play in life.

Being from the South, my paternal grandparents are extremely image conscious, and are always talking about weight and diet and comparing people. This was a normal conversation with them. My dad and I weren't very close, unfortunately. There was no emotional bond. He couldn't fully express himself and was tormented by his own internal struggles. He would pick on me calling me "massive." I think he was trying to be endearing, but it was hurtful. I think he thought he was being cute. He was smart, having taught for many years at a college and having a PhD in philosophy, but not in parenting. He was caught up in his own issues, and so our relationship was shallow and not good for me emotionally.

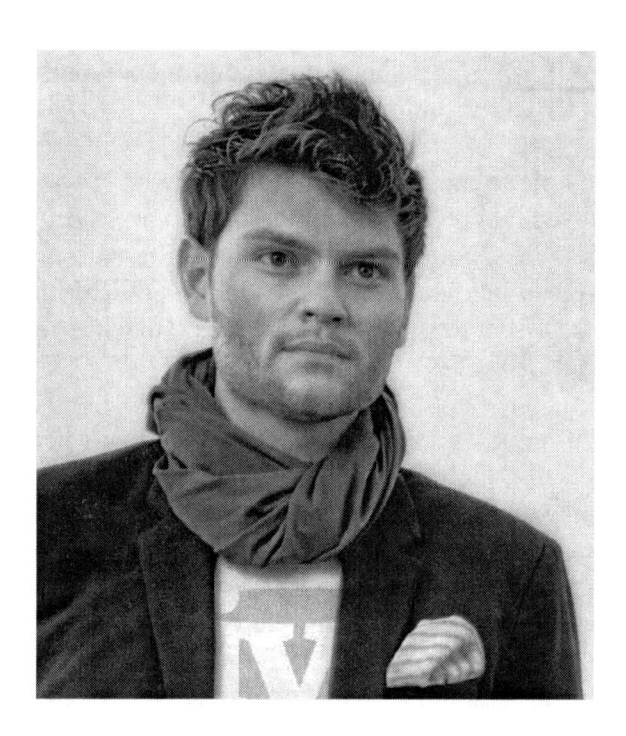

As I landed my first job, I wanted to build my image, self-esteem and confidence. I wanted to be more fashionable, more attractive and have more energy. I wanted to be stronger and step into who I truly knew myself to be and wanted to share with the world.

I had been researching different diets for years, like all fat people do. I knew a fair amount about nutrition from my Weight Watcher's days but felt like I needed something less conventional to help with the radical shift I wanted to create. I came across the HCG diet, read all about it, and researched it thoroughly. It seemed very interesting. I like stories and doing things that have stories and meaning attached to them. I'm drawn to provocative solutions and defying conventions.

The HCG diet is the brainchild of Dr. A Simeons. Human Chorionic Gonadotropin (HCG) is a hormone produced in pregnancy and is associated with weight loss. In combination with a very low, five hundred a day calorie diet, Dr. Simeons demonstrated great weight loss in many of his clients. There is an initial two-day "loading period" in which you are encouraged to fast load and eat large numbers of fat calories. Thereafter, you inject yourself (or take drops) daily of HCG for thirty days.

It seemed credible to me although not mainstream. I watched a lot of YouTube videos about people who had done it or were video-journaling their HCG journey. This seemed to be working for a lot of people. If you can be disciplined and stick to 500 calories a day and take the shots, it seemed like you could get amazing results. It was very economical, too.

So, when I started my career and moved to Dallas, where I knew no one, it seemed like the perfect time to start. I was there because the agency in Dallas was the best place for me at that stage of my career. It is the largest independent branding and creative agency in the US, a huge 600-person company with a long history of developing famous national brands. Stepping into my career, I wanted to simultaneously transform myself. I had my own apartment and was on my own for the first time. Working on myself was a priority.

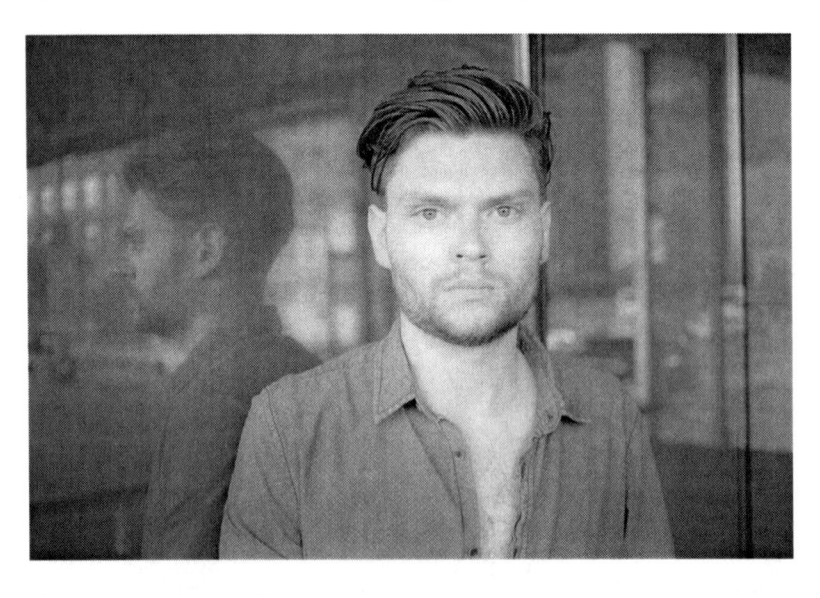

I downloaded Dr. Simeons' *Pounds and Inches* booklet and studied it. I ordered the HCG online, as well as the syringes I needed to inject myself. My first two days on the shots were loading days where I ate as much fat and as many calories as possible. It was fun!

I ate my worst favorite foods: a dozen Krispy Kreme donuts, chicken tenders, and lots of French fries. I gained five pounds.

I told everyone I knew that I was on this program. It worked exactly as I had read and witnessed on YouTube. On the 500 calories a day, I was losing about a pound a day, and I wasn't even hungry. I didn't have lots of energy, but I certainly was able to function in a sedentary lifestyle. I didn't do much socially but hang out by myself binge-watching TV and drinking green tea. Over the course of eight months, I lost 75 pounds.

I did everything by the letter. I took the required break after 30 days, to let my body reset. I was obsessive about keeping track of my food and really limiting myself to just five hundred calories daily. I weighed regularly. It was awesome watching my body change, to be able to get into clothes, even buy more fashionable ones.

I finally got to a really great weight. I felt proud of my accomplishment; I was successful, and I loved sharing my story. People were seeing my transformation before their eyes, and I was happy to give them the details and sing the praises of HCG.

I realize that the HCG diet is controversial but for me, that was part of the fun and the challenge. I had no adverse side effects. It changed my body chemistry and reliance on junk food. I think my stomach shrunk and my appetite shrunk, too. I don't have the taste for junk food and sweets that I used to. My meals are much simpler and healthier -- lean chicken breasts, fish, kale and other vegetables. I do go to restaurants and enjoy fine foods, but I'm not craving the same sorts of unhealthy convenience foods that I did before.

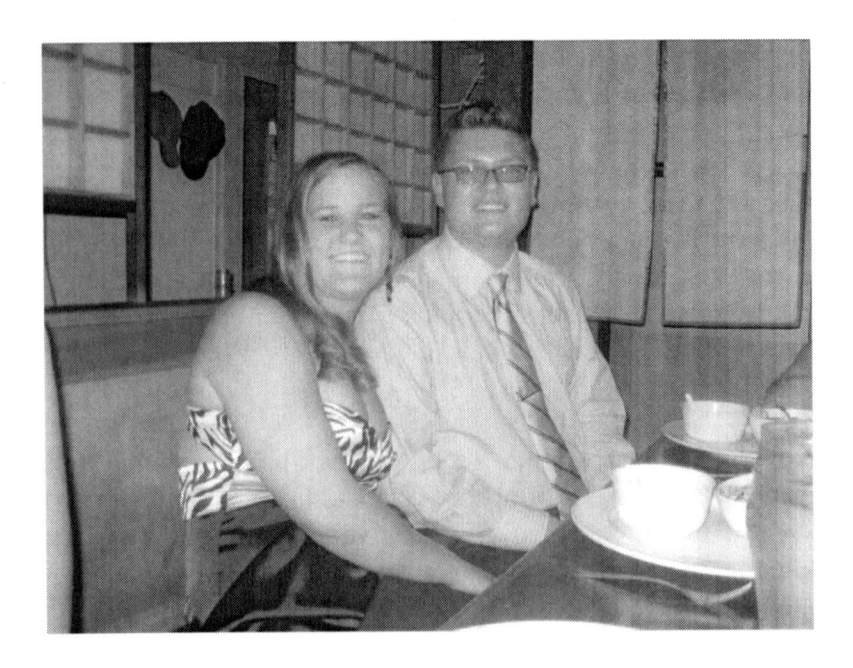

In February of 2012, another pivotal event happened. I moved to Santa Monica where I had taken another job. I was still on HCG then and eventually came off it three months later. In July, I joined a gym across from my work and hired a personal trainer -- it was a priority to get fitter and become stronger. The lifestyle in L.A. was much better than in Dallas, where I drove everywhere and the weather wasn't as conducive to outside activity.

I related much more to the Santa Monica lifestyle and people. I didn't have a car there, just a bike, which I rode along the Pacific Ocean bike path to my place of work on the Third St Promenade. Fortunate to have one of the most amazing commutes possible; I loved biking five miles a day. There were so many interesting people to interact with, plus the climate and the culture of fitness and exercise, all contributed to a much more active lifestyle. Of course, people there at the center of the entertainment industry, are very image conscious, and you don't want to stand out as an example of obesity or indolence. You want to look as good as everyone else does, like the actors and models.

The quality of food is also so much healthier. I got into the culture of juicing. My personal trainer was amazing and dedicated to my success. It was the first time in my life I could afford this support system. Her name was Jesse, and she was the head trainer at Burn Fitness right across the street from my office. I saw her two or three times a week for a year until I left for New York.

My objective was to improve my fitness, get lean and improve my overall health. I also did many group classes, from spin to TRX to yoga, as well as exercise with my roommates at the beach. I joined a kickball league. My company also organized beach volleyball games on a weekly basis, which were a lot of fun. They also threw a 21-day fitness challenge in which they hired a personal trainer who would provide daily lunchtime sessions, which again was great for fitness but also team bonding.

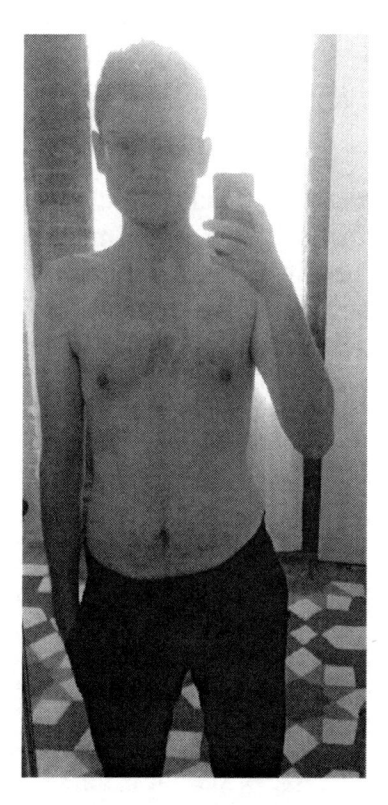

I lost 25 additional pounds over that year and decreased my BMI and body-fat percentage. I also went through several cycles of clothes. A new friend of mine, a fashion director, helped me completely redo my wardrobe!

I was living the LA lifestyle. I was even an impromptu model for one of my friends. I was happy! I felt as if I had come into my own professionally. My self-confidence increased along with my fitness. My body image was much improved.

So, it was a big upheaval leaving LA and heading to New York. Since I moved to New York, I have maintained my weight and fitness, although the culture is not as conducive to the level of activity in LA. I go to the Equinox gym in Midtown, but it's very different from the boutique gym in Santa Monica. The food quality in New York isn't as healthy, either. I walk a lot instead of bicycling. The weather isn't as conducive to outside activity; it's cold in the winter and too hot in the summer. But none of that has affected my fitness or my weight.

Because I lost my weight so quickly I have been overcoming 'body dysmorphia,' which means that despite my new weight and fitness level, I still mentally see myself as a big unattractive dude who didn't have anything to offer apart from professional success, smarts and energy. I didn't believe it when people indicated to me that they thought I was attractive.

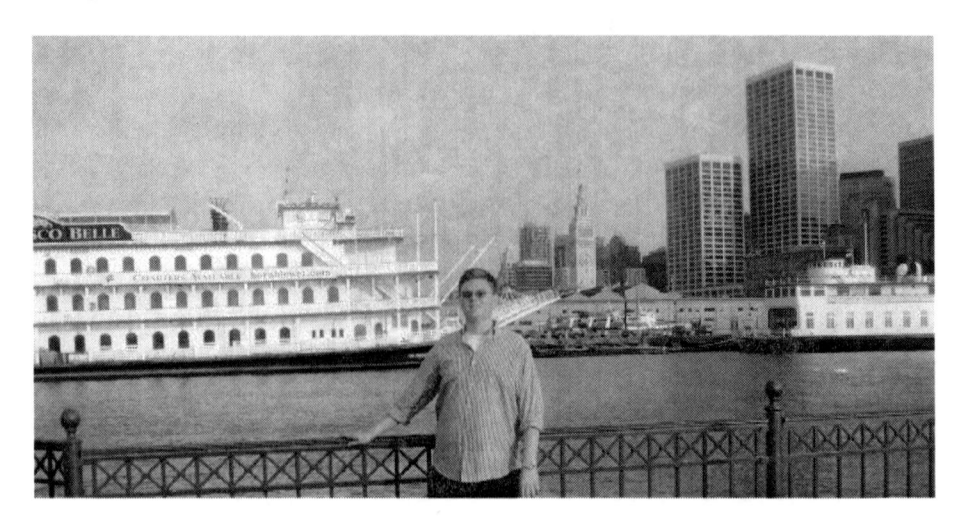

With time and continued positive reactions from others, I have made much progress transforming this negative perception about myself since coming to New York. For the first time in my life, I get the benefits of many compliments from friends and strangers. People don't believe it when I tell them that I have lost more than 100 pounds. I have maintained my weight at 156 pounds for well over a year.

The last relic of my old body is a bit of excess abdominal skin. I'm not sure how much I can change that through exercise or whether I'll ultimately need plastic surgery to remove it.

Being heavy is an emotional weight -- a negative constant. I've freed myself from that. Eating too much of the wrong stuff and being inactive makes your mood low, not necessarily clinically depressed, but just irritable and variable. I don't have those low moods any more.

My family isn't the best at acknowledgement -- they didn't encourage me along my journey, but they did and do compliment me. This has forced me to be dependent only on myself, to know that no one else was going to do it for me or even to expect help. I have a stronger sense of self having done it on my own. I am grateful in some ways that I had to work things out for myself. It helped me develop resilience and independence, and the deep knowing and satisfaction that I can create whatever I want in my life. And I am grateful that my family allowed me to follow my own path.

I am really curious and passionate about self-improvement and self-expression. In fact, I'm now a life coach practicing in the otological method. I love helping people shift their context to transform their lives and supporting them in their stand for what they want to create.

The genetic testing not only helped me on my weight loss journey it also erased my doubts about my Alzheimer's susceptibility. The disease has struck several members of my family, so it was a relief to discover that I do not have the predisposition or susceptibility to that form of dementia. Again, I would totally recommend this genetic testing service to anyone.

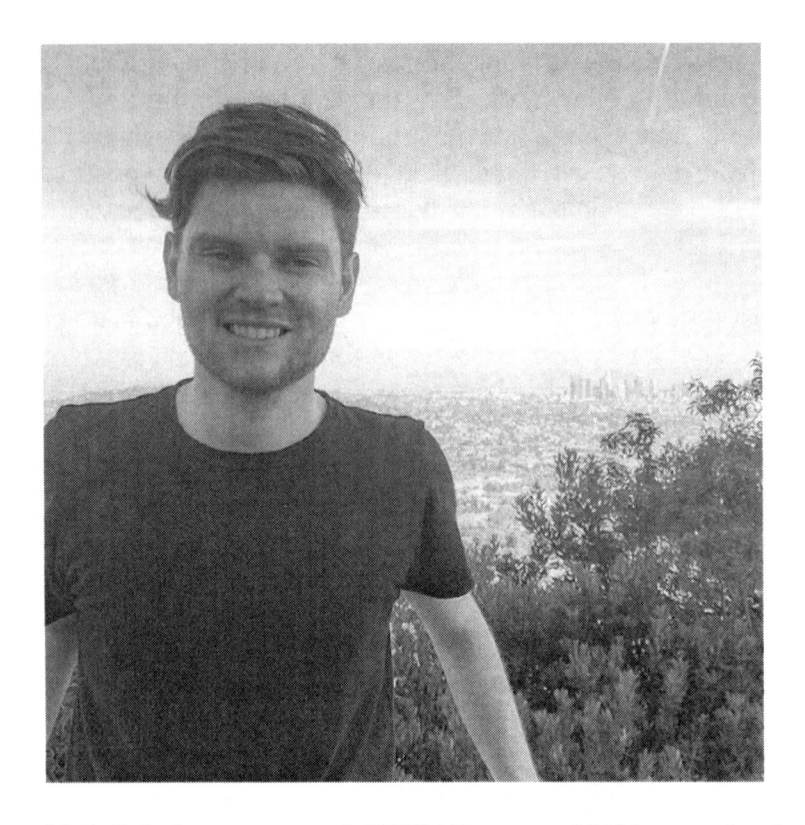

I would definitely recommend HCG if you are 100% committed and disciplined and set yourself up for success. No parties, no alcohol. Use this time to focus on yourself completely. A co-worker of mine in Santa Monica did it and was successful, losing 20 pounds in a short space of time. But weight loss doesn't occur in a vacuum. You need a vision of where you want to go in life and who you want to be. When you start achieving those goals, the positive feedback from the change will build your momentum, and you will achieve your dream.

I've always had a clear vision of my goals. I learned visualization techniques at Weight Watchers. When I was a teenager, I remember using visualization techniques to help me reach my school and career goals. I feel that being very specific and clear in my vision has worked personally as well as professionally. I am where I wanted to be, a strategist at an awesome branding firm, working on the most challenging and amazing projects for innovative brands.

Through my work, I really believe in manifestation science -- of setting a vision, declaring it to the world, and achieving it. When you do this, you never know how it will manifest, but it will if you welcome it and are open. I found HCG; I took the job in Santa Monica over another one in Raleigh, North Carolina; I found a personal trainer who is now a great friend. I'm doing the job I want at the smartest brand innovation firm in New York City. I've found that things work out when you set your mind to them and actively pursue your dreams.

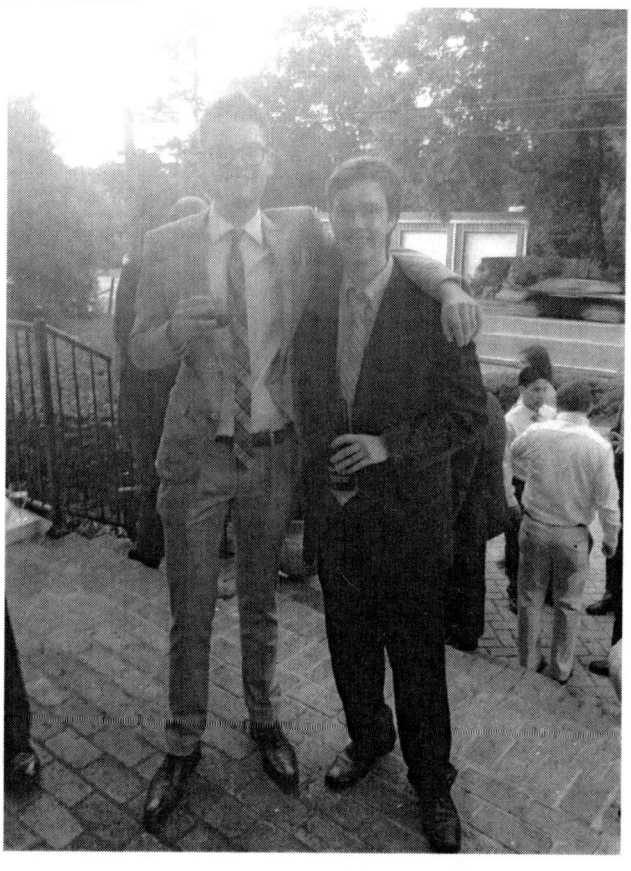

Part of ensuring that I manifest my dreams is surrounding myself with positive, supportive, like-minded people. They have been awesome influences and great mentors and examples. That's setting yourself up for success. Honestly, I don't think I could have achieved the same level of success in Atlanta.

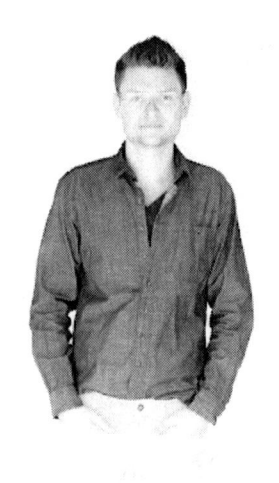

I had to step out of my comfort zone, leave everything that I knew to pursue what was possible for my life. Now I am 25, and this is just my start.

Charlene Barry

A Hike to the Top

In June of 2013 my friend Melissa, posted online that she was looking for anyone who was interested in going on a hike with her. I had stopped exercising for the previous three months, and this seemed like a great opportunity to get gently going again.

In the beginning of the year, I had started going to the gym with my husband and was making progress until I started to have severe pain in my right side. It didn't just hurt when I tried to work out, it hurt while I was sleeping, and randomly gave me trouble during the day. My doctor thought I might have a gallbladder problem, possibly as a result of my fat-laden past. He ordered some tests and when I went for the ultrasound, they poked and prodded me. It hurt so much I wanted to cry. I was advised to stop working out until they could come up with a diagnosis, so I had been sidelined. But eventually, over time, the pain subsided although it never went away completely.

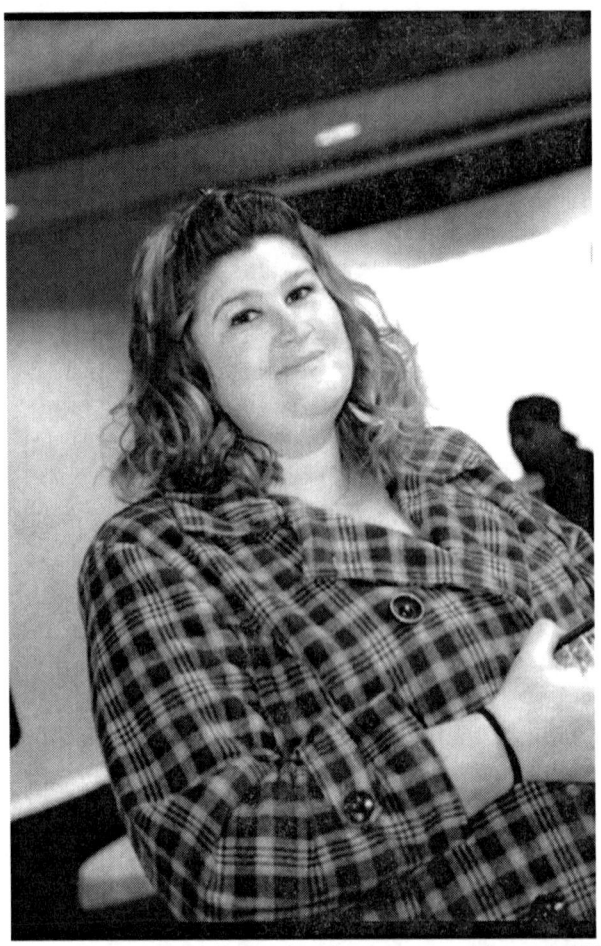

So, when I saw Melissa's hiking invitation, I told myself it was time to get up and get going. I needed to stop being lazy. We agreed to meet at an appointed time to hike in the woods near a mountain trail. I thought a leisurely walk in nature would be a good way to get back into some sort of physical activity. I bought a small water bottle with me and as much enthusiasm as I could muster.

We started out. I was dying after a mile. Melissa was good, though. She talked me through it. She distracted me, encouraged me and supported me. I huffed and I puffed. I moaned and I groaned. I occasionally cussed. But in the end I made it. I actually got to the top of the mountain! The leisurely walk in the woods turned out to be a five-mile hike up the mountain. I made it safely back in one piece in about three hours. I was sore. I was tired. I was surprised. But most of all, I was exhilarated.

That hike was wake-up call. If you told me beforehand that I was going to do that, I wouldn't have believed you, and I wouldn't have gone. But having made it to the top, I now realized that I can do anything I put my mind to.

The last few years of my life hadn't been ecstatic. In fact, for a lot of the time they had been downright depressing, as in 'I'm not sure I want to be around' depressing.
In 2007, I actually sat in a parking lot and with the car running, downed a lot of pills a professional at my college health center had given me. I got drowsy but I eventually made it home later, to my parent's home where I was living. My dad wanted to know whether the car was OK. Or that's how it seemed to me.

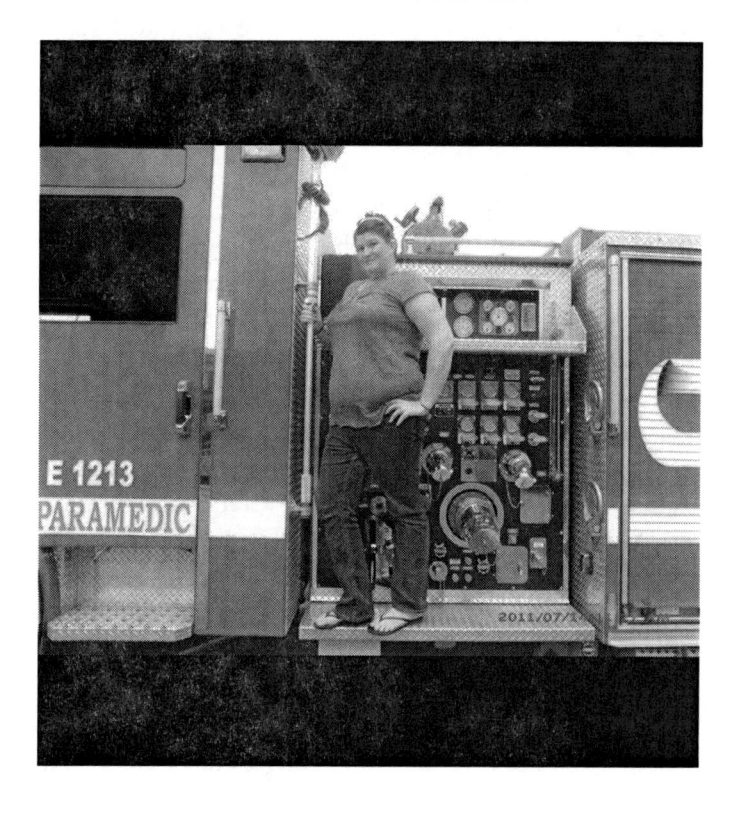

Growing up was difficult. When I was going through it and until my recent awakening, I did have some resentment, to be honest. I didn't feel as if I was loved. I didn't get much attention. What attention was available, such as it was, seemed to go to my older sister; life was hard. But it was for everyone and that all started long before I was born.

When my mom was a baby, my grandma was changing her diaper on an ironing board. The phone rang, and my grandmother answered it. As she did, my mom rolled off the ironing board and landed on her head. This led to a lifetime of epilepsy and other neurological issues, for which she has had brain surgery. My mom sometimes doesn't understand what's going on and there's definitely the feeling in our family that we all had/have to protect her and watch out for her. But she was able to get married and have two daughters. Not surprisingly perhaps, I, the younger one, am the ultimate caregiver. Mom's seizures were common while I was growing up, and I felt I always had to be there for her and my dad, not make any waves that might interfere with her brain waves and generally be as accommodating as possible.

My mom has also had heart problems, other health issues and was actually hit by a car in an accident that fractured one of her feet. But in addition to that, my parents simply aren't very demonstrative or outwardly affectionate. It's really hard to get an 'I love you' out of them. I think they do love me, but I have to assume it.

So, I have felt that I'm not good enough, and that I'm unlovable. I think I've finally figured out that I have been trying too hard to get love and attention. I've been in abusive relationships and stayed in them long after I realized it wasn't love or the way to get it. There have even been times when my parents have seen the abuse and not intervened or even said anything about it. Or that's how it seemed to me.

So, in 2009, after the break-up of another relationship in which I was bullied, called stupid and many other things that I can't write here, I once again had to return to living under my parent's roof. I sank into a huge depression. I didn't feel loved or comfortable. I didn't go to school. I didn't go to work. I thought of myself as disgusting.

One night I tried once again to seek oblivion with a bunch of pills and some incense oil. My dad actually checked in on me before going to bed. It was only when I called a friend of mine, someone who later turned out to be special to me, did anyone know what I had done.

I had dated this friend very briefly before breaking it off with him to pursue the renewal of a former relationship. But we stayed friends, and I trusted him enough to call him and tell him what I had done. He called 911, and the emergency services showed up at three in the morning and took me to the hospital to have my stomach pumped. A few months later, we started dating and in 2011, we got married.

It's clear looking back now at these times; I didn't care enough about myself. It was easier to take care of others because not only did that distract me from myself; it held the illusion that I was going to be really appreciated for being such a caring person. I know I wouldn't do that again, and I know I will not go back to the depression and the suicidal feelings. I feel good about finally taking care of myself.

Looking back, I wasn't really overweight at all until the fourth grade. In fact, I was downright skinny up until that time. It was as if I just suddenly grew at the age of 10. In fact, I did grow taller. In middle school, I weighed around 190 and was about 5'7". I gained another thirty pounds or so while in high school. By the time I left high school, I was 5'11" and 216.

Sometimes as a child, I had to play the role of my mom. I couldn't have a normal conversation with her as she doesn't understand, so it is really tough to communicate with her. My poor dad has to deal with a lot. We don't really talk about it. When I did want to talk about the dynamic in the family and how we felt, my sister nixed it -- or more accurately objected, and I backed off. I didn't really have a mentor. Then I went into counseling when I got to college.

The first few counselors weren't helpful at all. They mostly just gave some pills. Then I had another one who would always be late or run over with the previous appointment and generally cut my time, which really annoyed me. Just what a person starving for attention needs -- a therapist who doesn't give them the time or show them respect! I did finally find a counselor whom I liked very much. She wanted to bring my parents in for a joint session, which I was all up for. But then I lost my insurance, and it never happened.

I did okay in high school. I was an average student. I did have friends but limited my social activity because dad would say 'no' -- we were restricted for money and time, and I didn't want to bother them. My mom could have seizures at any time but often at night. Even now she has a couple a week. Somebody needs to be there.

When I started college at Cal State San Marcos I was, of course, living with my parents. Honestly, I was struggling, gaining weight and just trying to find someone who cared about me. Before long, I moved in with a boyfriend. I was also working full-time in a retail job in the mall, as well, of course, going to school. It was a mess. I was a mess. My aunt and uncle helped pay for college but when I got an F in algebra, they started to compare me with my sister. I did care about my studies even though it might have seemed like I didn't. I just didn't care about myself and proved it by staying in an abusive relationship for two years. He cheated; I kept going back.

I know now that I'm worth more than that. That is not love, and I can't tolerate that. I went back and forth between my retail job, other jobs and school, as well as different mood states. I did finally get my bachelor's degree in social science. It took me a grand total of eight years. When I was going through that really difficult phase with my mood, energy and self-esteem, I dropped out of everything and then had to convince my employers, and my college, that I was ready to return. But I hung in there, and I made it.

I wanted to be a special-education teacher but found my way to helping adults with disabilities. Me, in the helping profession? Go figure. I'm an administrator-in-training for the facility I work for. I have all my certifications and hope soon to be promoted officially into that position. Honestly, it is only recently that I realize how strong my co-dependency and need to get validation through helping others really is. People I use to date have disabilities, including my husband. I work as a caregiver in home for adults with disabilities. I didn't really appreciate how strong a dynamic that has been for me. Not until I climbed that mountain, in fact. My fitness and weight loss journey increased my self-awareness. It wasn't until I was actually doing it, that I could realize how much I had neglected my own needs.

I still struggle with drawing appropriate boundaries. I gave up a friendship because I realized it was unbalanced and everything I was putting in was not getting reciprocated. And until 2013, I was not doing anything about my weight. I didn't care. I didn't think about my body. I knew I was in trouble. I knew I had to do something about it but never did. Even when I got married in 2011, I didn't care about how I looked or whether I could even fit in my dress. But, I'm happy to report that all that has changed. I take pride in myself now. I want to look in the mirror.

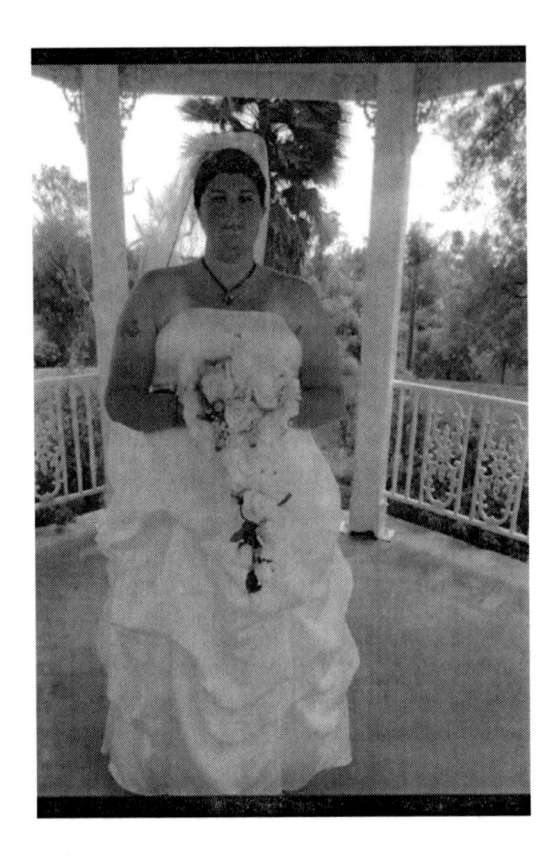

So, at the beginning of 2013, my husband and I joined a gym and started working out together. But I was still drinking too many sodas and probably too much alcohol on occasion. Then I got hurt. Then I climbed that mountain.

After that first fateful hike, I started to hike on my own as well as add some of my own aerobics. I also joined myfitnesspal and the program really increased my awareness. It tells you the balance of the foods you're eating as well as calories. I stopped all sodas and other sugary drinks, cut down on the alcohol and basically drank water. I was much more vigilant with my eating, and within a few weeks I had dropped fourteen pounds.

At the end of July, I also joined TOPS, a weight loss group, for added support and especially accountability. The accountability that the group provided has helped me stay focused on my ultimate goal. They have kept me motivated through it all.

I developed a regimen where I was hiking, going to the park to run and going to the gym. I lost weight -- between one and two pounds -- for ten consecutive weeks. When I actually gained a little in the eleventh week, I wasn't fazed at all. I knew it was natural fluctuation, and I lost three pounds the next week.

By September of 2013, I was working out six days a week. I lost a little focus during the holiday season but soon picked it up again. When I'm at the gym now I start at 6am. I do an hour on the treadmill at a steep incline and then the circuit, which consists of ten weight exercises and ten step workouts. I push myself and sometimes it seems a bit much. But I also get mad at myself if I miss a workout.

Nutritionally, I eat 1590 calories when I'm not exercising and up to 2000 when I am.

For breakfast, I typically have the same things in one combination or another: yogurt, protein bar, fruit, and oatmeal. Lunch is similar, with the addition of a fiber bar. For snacks, I have an apple or other fruit. My husband usually cooks dinner: chicken, meat, fish with vegetables. There are some days when I don't eat that much during the day, and I want a bigger evening meal, but I really try to eat-- and drink -- healthily now.

Some days my energy is up and some days it's not. I work hard, and I exercise hard. When I'm tired, the support group helps because I know they are there and waiting, and I don't want to let the team down. Myfitnesspal really helps me keep track by breaking my exercise and nutrition down so I can see what I'm doing. If I'm nutritionally off course, it's that I'm not having enough protein. Sugar is my biggest struggle. I'm not a white foods -- bread, rice, pasta -- person, but I crave chocolate all the time.

I deal with the sugar issue by having small amounts, typically about 90 calories, usually frozen fruit and a little ice-cream. That way, I can have a little sweet fix, but I don't overdo it. We did buy some Girl Scout cookies, and I consider it a major victory that one of the boxes sat around the house unopened for four months! That's a sign that I now have more control, because previously, I would eat one whole box in a short sitting.

My husband and I just moved back in with parents about a year or so ago. They are having a hard time, and we moved in to help them out. My parents are actually very supportive. They will tell me what a great job I'm doing. My habits are also rubbing off on them.

My dad has heart problems and is scheduled for heart valve replacement. He walks with me in the park. He is definitely eating better and recently told me he lost ten pounds. Mom is even moving around more, walking around the block during the day. I think I've helped them through my own example.

My husband is still a Pepsi addict and occasionally has cookies around the house. On the other hand, he reminds me all the time how much he loves me and how beautiful I am. He will call or text me during the day to support me, to nurture me and to cherish me.

I've got him involved in my exercise, too. He walks with me, and we do events together. I continue to really enjoy the hiking. I really enjoy the alone time, the opportunity to get away, to meditate in nature. There's a trail that goes almost to the top of Mount Woodson. At the top, there's something called Potato Chip rock, because, well, it looks like a potato chip. There's a huge rocky overlook there, which is kind of scary but also a testament to the achievement. It's an eight-mile loop, and I love doing it -- being able to do it. I could never have imagined myself being able to do that. It gives me confidence and hope. It makes me feel that I can achieve things.

I feel that I am achieving things that I wasn't doing or not seeing before. As I've mentioned, I work serving adults (ages 18-59) with developmental disabilities. I work with those who have impairments but are functional. Part of my job involves going to their homes to deliver programs and services. I help then with everything: meds, daily activities, laundry, doctors' appointments, hygiene, retraining maladaptive behaviors-- everything. I'm also currently helping to start up a day program.

I enjoy it but I have to admit some days are tough and frustrating. But then one of my clients will do something extraordinary, and I will get so excited. For example, recently a client who barely speaks actually said, "can I have some juice, please?" I couldn't believe it! It was awesome. I was jumping up and down; I was so excited!

I'm impressed that many of my clients put so much into life and yet enjoy the simple things. They have awesome personalities and outlooks. My work is never the same, and it's always a reminder of the blessings that I have.

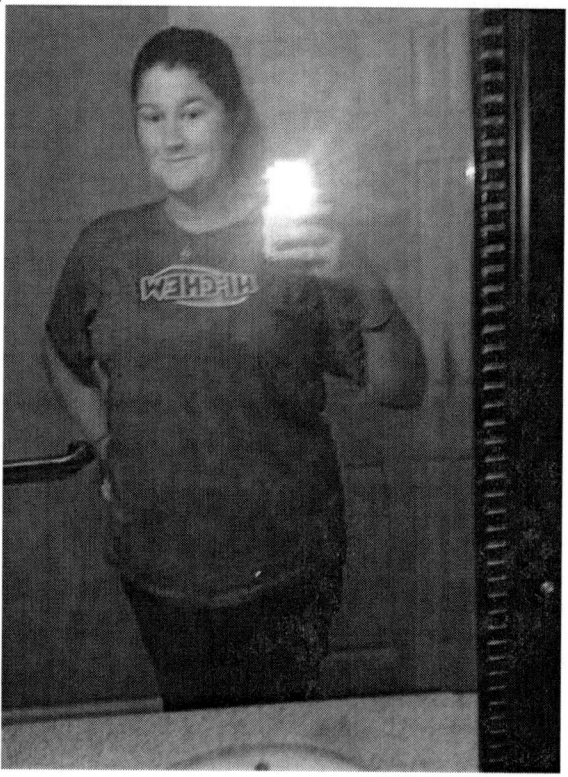

I'm now at 214, and I have lost 51 pounds. I want to get to 165 for a hundred-pound loss in total. My doctor says I don't need to lose that much, but that is what I am going to do.

I am a monkey fanatic. Ever since I was little, I've loved monkeys. My parents gave me monkey dolls and stuffed animals all the time when I was a child. If I could, I would have a real one. We now even have 'Monkey Business' awards at work and when my boss goes out of town, she often brings me back monkey-related souvenirs. I've even thought about working with them, but it's my sister who studied zoology, and anyway I prefer my current job. I think it's the energy, the impishness, the fun that monkeys suggest that appeals to me -- all things I didn't really have myself until the last few months.

I may have some ways to go, but I think I have finally found myself. Strange to say, I found myself at the top of a mountain. On a peak, surrounded by beauty, and nature -- and God.

I should tell you that I grew up in a Christian home but went off His path when I hit fifteen and stopped going to church altogether by the time I was eighteen. Then, after my last suicide attempt-- as well promising my family I would never do anything like that again.-- I made the same promise to God. I told myself I'd get a tattoo to remind me of that promise and how much God loved me. I didn't do it immediately. But when we moved back into my parents' home in 2012, I could feel the depression coming on again, so I finally got the tattoo to remind me of His infinite love for me.

It still took me a year to finally love myself as much. He and everyone else in my life loves me. That's when I started going back to church. And so when I work out, it's my fellowship with God that drives me. The only music I listen to is either worship music or Christian rock. Today, he reminded me how much I need Him. A song came on called "Strong Tower." Some of the lyrics are "you are my strong tower" and "I will run to your mountain." And, guess what? The place I hike is a mountain with a tower. So I really do think that's why I love this place so much because it reminds me of His beauty, and it's where I spend a lot of time in fellowship with Him.

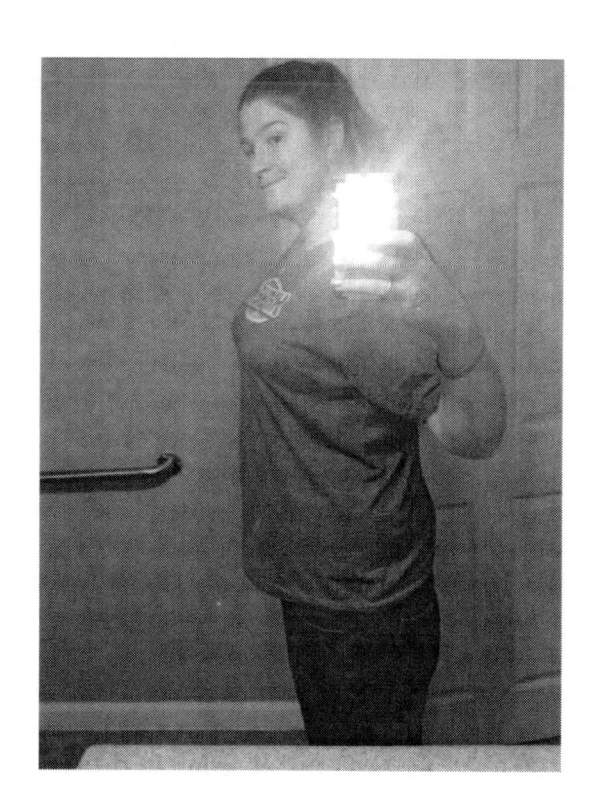

Alexa Fredericks

Fructose Down, Energy Up

Until I was seven years old, I was pretty active. I had some friends, and we used to play outside a lot. But then they moved away and all that stopped, and I found myself more and more inside and inactive. Another event happened during that time -- my mom opened her own salon and day spa in 2001. She was frequently working, and it was hard to spend a lot of time together. I think it was tough for me. So, by the time I was in middle school, I was unhappy with my weight and my body.

I lived with my parents and my mom's parents, and all of them in one way or other had some health issues. And some of those health problems had a big influence on my decision to focus on my weight.

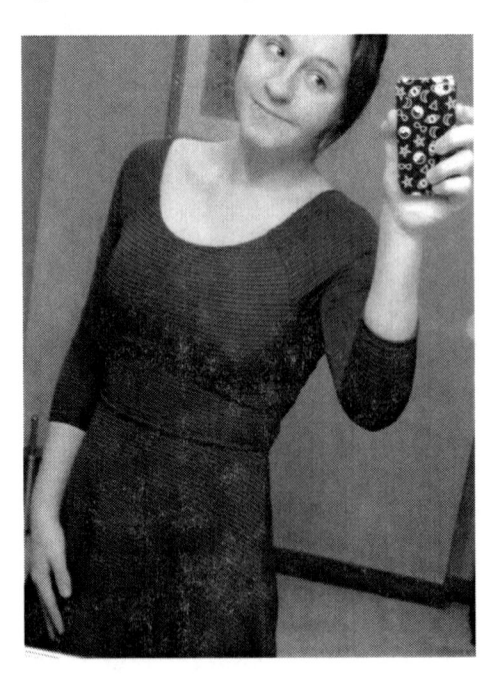

At one point, my dad was overweight and a heavy smoker, but he got his act together. It was my mom and her parents that gave me the greatest cause for concern. Both my mother's parents are overweight and diabetic.

My grandparents are both from Italy. Enough said. They are both diabetic. They are able to manage their diabetes now, but I know they both wish they could still enjoy a lot of the foods they used to eat but can no longer. Seeing my grandparents miserable, at first, during their sudden diet changes, made me realize I did not want to be faced with the same issue in the future and that motivated me to be more cautious and concerned.

However, there was another family health issue that was even more important and influential on my thinking.

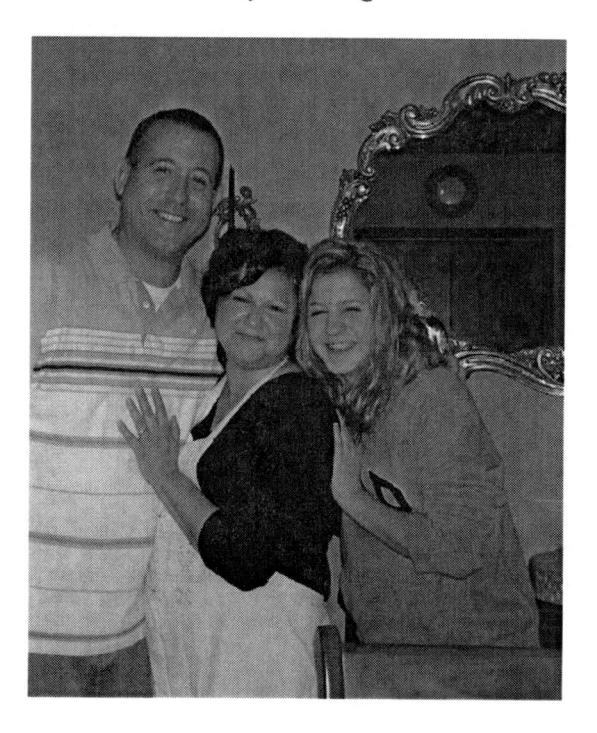

When I was twelve years old, I discovered I had a blood clotting disorder called 'factor five Leiden' (sometimes written as 'factor V Leiden'). It is basically a disease which causes thickening of the blood. My mom also has it. She had me tested when her doctor told her the disease was hereditary. Diet and exercise play a huge role in the condition. Being inactive and overweight can increase the possibility of getting a blood clot. I have to be aware of foods that contain vitamin K and limit my intake of them because they are natural blood thickeners. Vitamin K is found in many vegetables like green beans, spinach, asparagus, and lettuce. There is medication for the condition, but I couldn't go on it until I was eighteen. And on the subject of family history and vascular disease, my mom's dad has also had a stroke.

Fortunately, I have not yet experienced a blood clot and hope to continue living healthier so I do not experience any in the future. However, you can imagine that discovering I had this condition was motivating for me. It took a few months for the seriousness of it to sink in, but I really started to get motivated about my weight and my health as I was heading into high school. It was then that I made a conscious effort to change my lifestyle.

In fairness, my parents and others wanted me to be in sports all along. Mom had played softball and dad had played basketball; they both wanted me to play some type of sport and be active. But I really didn't get involved. Gym class was miserable. Mom, in particular, kept pressing me to find some sort of sport. But I always found some excuse. I felt uncomfortable most of the time. I never was happy with what I was wearing and knew it wasn't my clothes; it was me.

When I got to high school, I did become more active. For one thing, the building was big and four stories tall and to be honest I sometimes had a hard time getting to the right class on time. It was difficult climbing all those stairs. I was 5'2" tall and weighed 158.

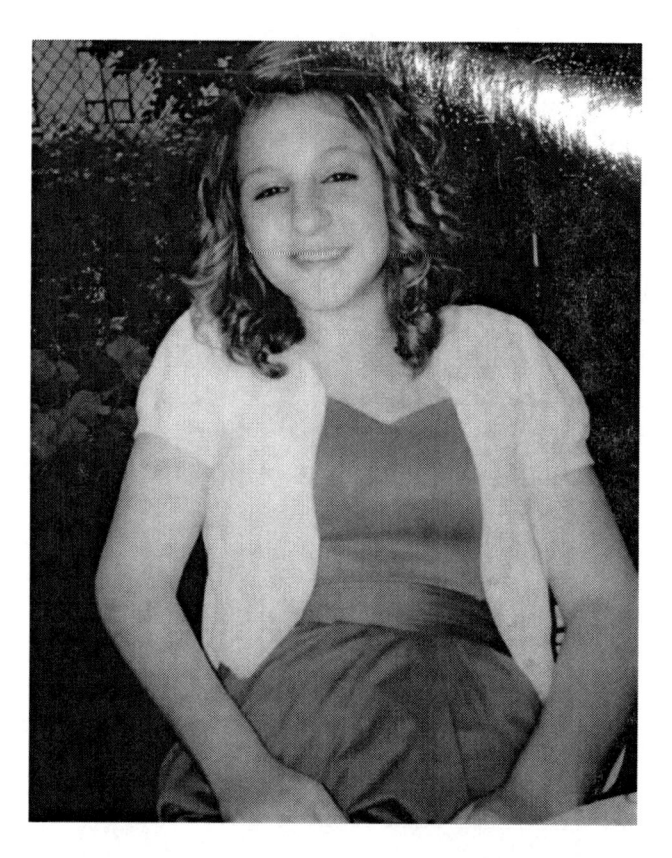

For a while, I did participate in an early morning running group. But I quit after a month as it didn't seem to be making a difference. I guess I was expecting magic results. This was a pattern for me back during most of my high school years. I wanted the weight to come off fast. So I often exercised for a couple of weeks then convinced myself there was no difference; I "took a break," also known as "quitting."

The next quick fix came when I discovered that a friend of mine was Vegan. I thought that was the magic answer, and so, I went on a vegan diet for a while. On this diet, I ate a majority of vegetables each day mixed into salads. I tried smoothies and vegan pastas as well. I was not a huge fan of the vegan diet and surprise, surprise; it didn't last very long. For a while, I felt pretty good, but I did not notice any weight loss from eating this way -- and weight loss was my main goal. I quit after a month. I was still eating too many calories. On the Vegan diet, I often felt tired as well and later discovered that not eating meat was the main cause of my fatigue.

High school was really difficult for me at first. I had low self-esteem and wasn't motivated to do a lot. I would definitely admit to being lazy, for the most part. Sitting home and watching television was much easier than exercising or even trying to make friends, but even that got boring very quickly. Around my junior year, I started talking to more people and getting out, and I felt more confident, generally. My parents and teachers pushed me a little at a time to try new things, like playing basketball after school and doing volunteer work. Slowly and surely, I made new friends and became more active.

But my weight still bothered me a lot towards the end of high school. Then one thing critical happened.

I started dating.

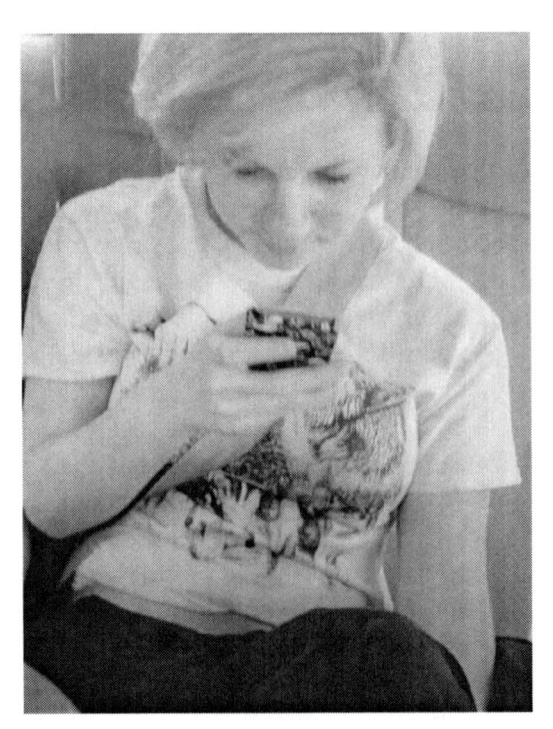

My boyfriend Lane was very supportive. He wasn't judgmental but he wasn't passive either, just supportive, and he encouraged me to do lose weight for myself. For me, not anyone else. Then he joined Marines. We still keep in touch as much as possible through phone calls and video chats today because he is constantly traveling. We try to visit one another at every chance we get.

I had attended summer school for three years in high school, and as a result I was able to graduate at 17. After graduation, I did try to step up my exercise. I adopted a dog, Bella a Pekinese and, of course, started to walk her regularly. I also started to walk with my parents on a trail behind our house. I went on another diet with my dad where we replaced meat with fish. And, significantly, we focused on cutting down on the carbs.

One thing I noticed about eating carbs, was that the more carbs I ate-- especially the high glycemic carbs-- the less energy I had. I now know that for me, as with a lot of other people, eating these foods overloads my blood with glucose, and that's what makes me feel sluggish. Then, when my energy was low, I thought the answer was to eat more carbs, and the cycle continued. I think it affected my energy a lot -- even to the point of being so sluggish in the morning that I really couldn't -- or didn't want to -- get up.

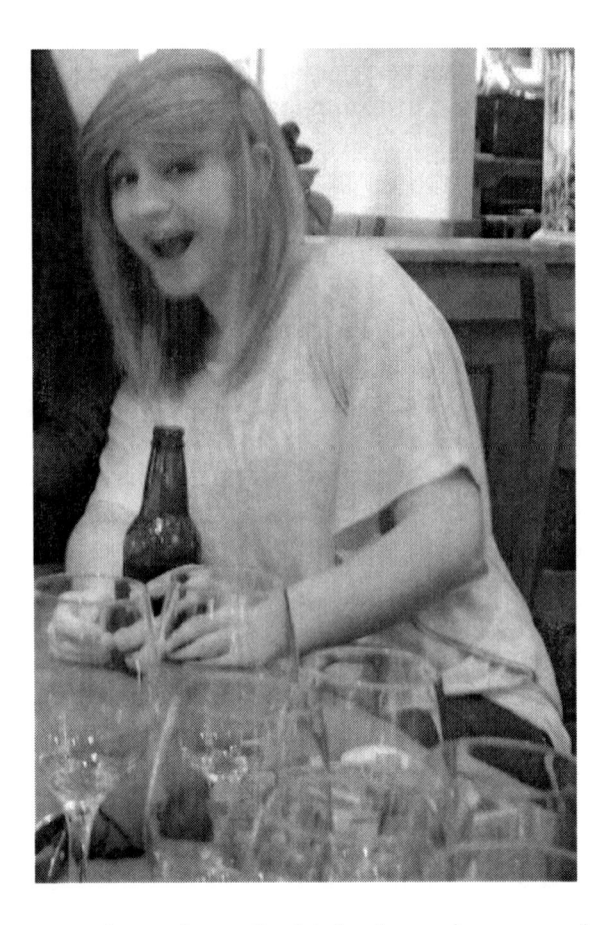

Cutting down on the carbs -- the high glycemic ones -- has been the key. I now know the difference between the high glycemic carbs, like bread, pasta and sodas, and the less glycemic ones like fruits and vegetables. In the bread and pasta and sodas, (the high-fructose corn syrup ones) the fructose is "free fructose" and is therefore, much more highly concentrated and absorbed into the blood stream. The vegetable and fruit fructose is tied to fiber and far less is absorbed. Moreover, what is absorbed is taken in much more slowly, so you don't get an overload of glucose in your blood.

Now that I have continued to cut down on those foods dramatically I have a lot more energy. And with more energy has come motivation. I mentioned above that I used to find it hard to get up in the morning. Not anymore! And previously even though I was tired I didn't sleep very well. Now I get a solid six hours. I'm now more a night owl, but I am no longer sluggish.

There are several ways I have cut out the 'free fructose.' I used to eat a lot of bread and sandwiches and have now cut that out almost completely. If I have anything like that, I have vegetable wraps from my local import grocery store.

I also used to drink a lot of sodas, but they have lost their appeal. And I've learned that sodas are as big a problem as foods because of the "free fructose" they contain. Now it's water and water-based drinks. Breakfast is typically fruit and yogurt.

There are a couple of things that I do now that also make a big difference.

I eat slower now. This allows me to stop before I am completely full. I always used to eat until I was stuffed but by eating slower I can stop when I am comfortably full, not just stuffed. The fact is that it takes a good twenty minutes for the stretch in your stomach to signal the brain to stop eating. If you don't pay attention, your body will allow you to eat until you are stuffed.

I also have small snacks throughout the day, so I don't get hungry. Those snacks are granola bars, fruit, salads, and veggie wraps -- no free fructose. I also learned that lean meats are definitely great for you and give you lots of energy. Freezing fruit is helpful; frozen blueberries taste like ice-cream to me and help me stay away from the real thing.

And one other tactic really helped. For one month I kept a detailed food journal. This made me much more aware about how much I was eating. So, with the combination of greater awareness and energy and getting off the glucose merry-go-round, I developed more control over my eating. That gave me more energy, which led to more motivation, and put me in a positive spiral, that helped me lose thirty-five pounds, which I have kept off for a year.

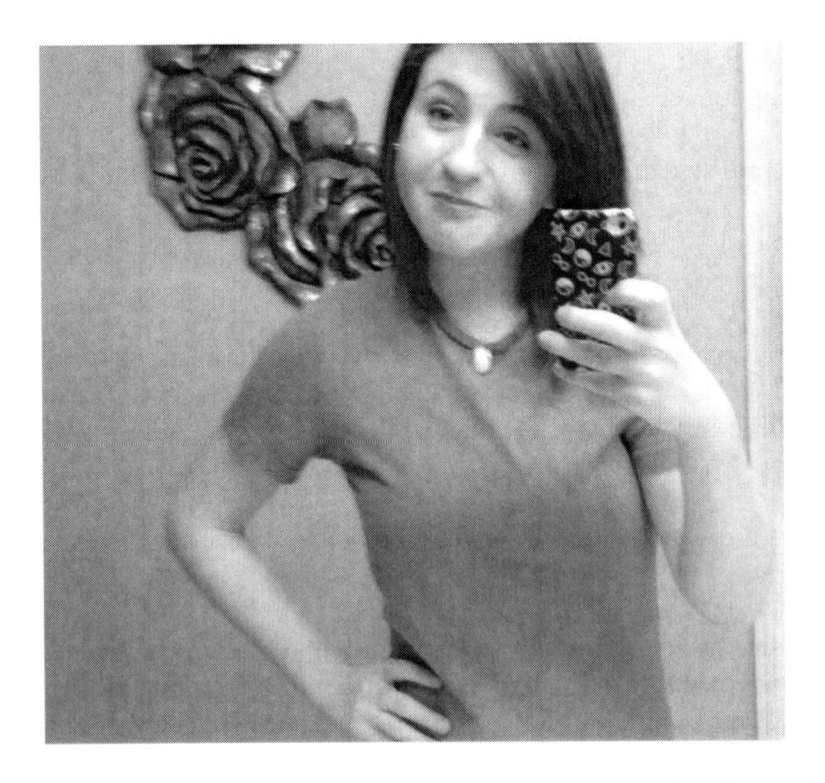

Another thing that helped me lose the weight and keep it off -- eating out way less often. The fact is that when you eat out, you are much more likely to have the carbs and the free fructose. Eating at home really helped me cut back on the glucose habit that was so necessary for me to get out of my nutrition rut. As far as eating at home is concerned, I am lucky because my grandfather enjoys gardening and grows all sorts of vegetables. My grandmother makes home-made tomato sauce and says things like, "You're Italian so just eat!" That's okay. The home-made tomato sauce doesn't have fructose in it like it probably would if I were eating it at a restaurant.

All this energy also helped me become more active. I started to work out with my dad in our home gym. (Yes, I now actually use it.) I run about four miles regularly. I also swim. I have also become an assistant coach at the high school for different activities and levels. The girls are non-judgmental, and it keeps me feeling young!

Running has helped me the most. Playing basketball and volleyball with friends also made exercise more fun for me. The only exercise technique I was never really fond of, was yoga. I do enjoy meditation, but yoga was difficult for me. I felt like I was not achieving much, and it was too slow-paced for me.

There have been many benefits of my weight loss and continued maintenance.

I used to wear sweat pant clothes but several months ago I started investing in a new wardrobe. It was weird to get new clothes. I'm down three sizes. It was a bit uncomfortable at first, but now I love it!

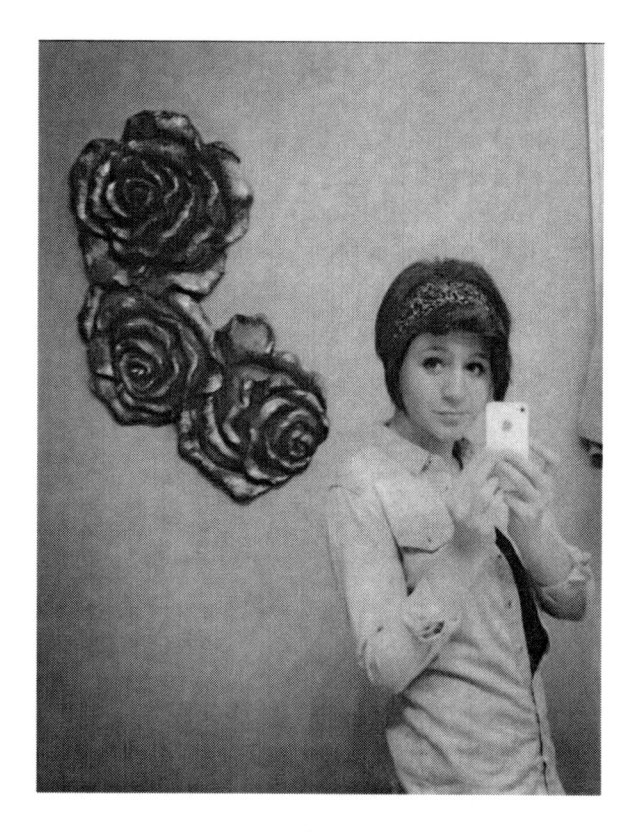

I also have a good group of girlfriends, and we confide and support each other. I'm much more confident in my own skin.

With my new-found confidence, I've been considering different careers. I have seriously considered an army career. It would be a cool adventure. Apart from my boyfriend in the Marines, my favorite teacher was in the army. Currently, I am taking law enforcement courses at college.

Being positive and staying motivated helped the most, but those are functions of the increased energy I have, as a result of avoiding free fructose and exercising. Sure, I have days where I would rather stay inside on the couch than go jogging, but I know I cannot make a habit of that. Now and then I'll have breaks, but I keep in mind that I'm happy weight-wise where I am and want to stay this way. That motivates me to keep going.

So, my advice is never try to rush weight loss. Each person has his or her own diet and exercise expectations that work for them. Certainly get off those high glycemic foods to see whether that will make the difference for you that it did for me. Do what makes you comfortable and find a healthy routine that works best just for you. Be consistent and don't expect overnight results. Everything takes time but is surely worth it.

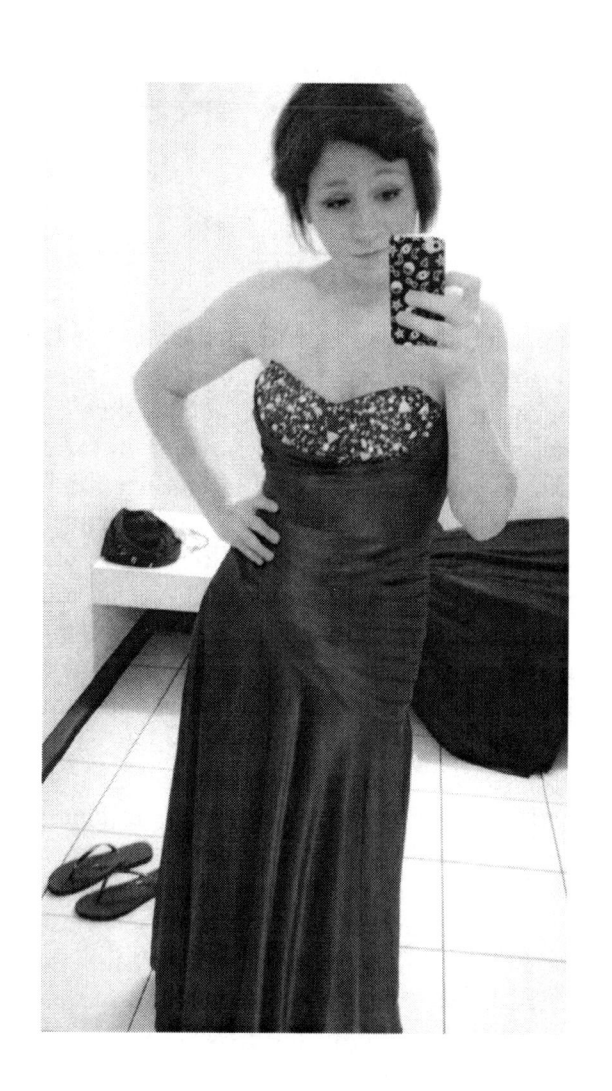

Katie Petersen

No End Date

I was so excited I couldn't sleep, or that's the way I felt when I woke up at 5 o'clock in the morning. It was going to be a great day, a day to celebrate being an American. I was happy that my parents had decided to come on this trip with me. I travel a lot for work and have a lot of frequent-flier miles and I kept telling my mom and dad that they should come with me on some of my trips. Finally, they decided that they would make this trip with me. So here we were, the family from rural Minnesota, in Washington D.C. And today, we were going to take a tour of the White House. It was September 11, 2001.

We were scheduled to take the 8:15 am tour, but now I was wide awake and raring to go. I convinced my somewhat sleepy parents; we should get there as soon as possible. We excitedly got ourselves ready and showed up at Pennsylvania Avenue in plenty of time. We arrived early so we could get in on the 7:45 tour. The tour was fantastic, and I felt a real connection to our heritage.

When it was over, we left and were at the Washington Monument when it happened. The ground shook, a terrible rumble that seemed like an earthquake, and in the distance; we could see smoke coming from the area near the Pentagon. Suddenly, there were police everywhere. It sounded like a hundred sirens went off at once, a surreal sound that gives me goose-bumps to this day. What's happening? No one seemed to know. The police came up to us and asked if we knew what was going on. No. "They've hit the Twin Towers, and we're advising everyone to get the hell out of town."

Who were "they"? What is happening?

While this was going on, in a plane-- over farmland not unlike our own, in Pennsylvania-- some brave Americans decided to take matters into their own hands. As a result, United Airlines flight 93 came down in a field in Shanksville, Pennsylvania and not in the White House a few minutes later -- at exactly the time my parents and I were scheduled to be there.

We headed back to the hotel. Just before we got there, we could see fighter jets overhead, an awesome sight. We have an Air National Guard near us in Sioux Falls, and I've seen fighters flying overhead many times. But this was surreal. This was for real.

We watched the television every minute of that incredible day, like everyone else. We eventually left Washington and visited some relatives, before making it back home, safe and sound, via Baltimore.

I'd like to tell you that awed by this combination of circumstances, I got my act together and finally addressed the problem of the extra one hundred plus pounds I was carrying. It's not that simple. The personal impact of that day was going to be significant, but it would be a delayed reaction not an instantaneous one.

At this point in my life, in my mid-twenties, I was pretending that all was well. It wasn't but I am, or was, a very good pretender. I was the one who always had a smile on her face but some unrecognized pain in my heart. I had been like that for most of my life. The helper. The pleaser. The caretaker -- of everyone else that is. I was a great friend.

I was born to two loving parents who worked hard on their farm. I had a brother who was two years older than me. The farm kept us all very active. There were always things that needed doing and there was always food on the table. Most of it was home-grown and "clean." There was plenty of meat, potatoes and vegetables. Perhaps we ate a bit too much of it but we certainly worked off a lot of those calories. My mother had a few weight issues, and she was constantly aware of weight -- especially for us girls in the family. Truth be told, my brother, was a little overweight too. Dad wasn't.

It wasn't long; however, before I developed another problem. I grew tall. Very tall. In fact, I was easily the tallest girl in my pre-school and elementary classes. It didn't help that while I was tall, the classes were small, so I stood out much more than I might have done in a bigger class where there might have been other girls close to my height.

Occasionally, I would be teased by my other eleven classmates, but I wasn't really self-conscious about my weight until the fifth grade. I was very athletic, very sociable and the teasing was mostly good-natured. I labeled myself as "the fat funny one," to survive and occasionally, in darker moments, I thought of myself as "the monster."

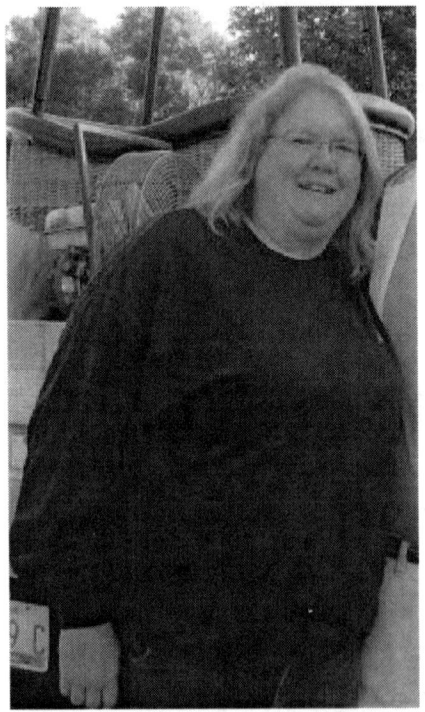

But by the time I was in middle school I had become a lot more self-conscious, even though, finally, one of my classmates had finally got to be as tall as I. I was much more aware, and not just about my height and weight. I mean conscious about me. As a person. And another event happened during that time that rocked my world.

I remember it very clearly. It was a Saturday and mom was getting ready to go to work, a part-time job she had. She was coming down the stairs and felt dizzy. She became unsteady on her feet. Grandpa called the ambulance and then drove my mom to a nearby town to meet the paramedics. She was immediately transferred to a hospital in Sioux Falls.

By the time my brother and I got to the hospital, it had been determined that my mom had had a mild stroke. I was worried but it certainly could have been worse. It looked like she was going to be fine. Before I got to see her again, however, she'd had a massive stroke. If she hadn't been in the hospital, she would have almost certainly died, according to the doctors. She was only 34.

When I went to see my mom in the hospital the next day, I was overwhelmed. She was now in the Intensive Care Unit attached to all sorts of monitors and machines. Even as I think about that scene today, I still get emotional. It was clear to this 11-year-old girl, that her mom was in serious trouble. And if she was in serious trouble, so was I.

My mother was in the hospital for fully two months before she was released. As the dutiful, loving daughter, there wasn't anything I wouldn't do to make the situation better for my mother, my dad and my brother. I quickly stepped up into the care-giving role and took on some of the family roles that my mom couldn't yet do. That meant more time in the kitchen as my mom coached me in how to make some of the family favorites. I also did a lot of the cleaning and generally helping my mom who was still severely restricted in her activities. I also learned how to shop because sometimes there wasn't time for cooking, and we had to fall back on food from the stores.

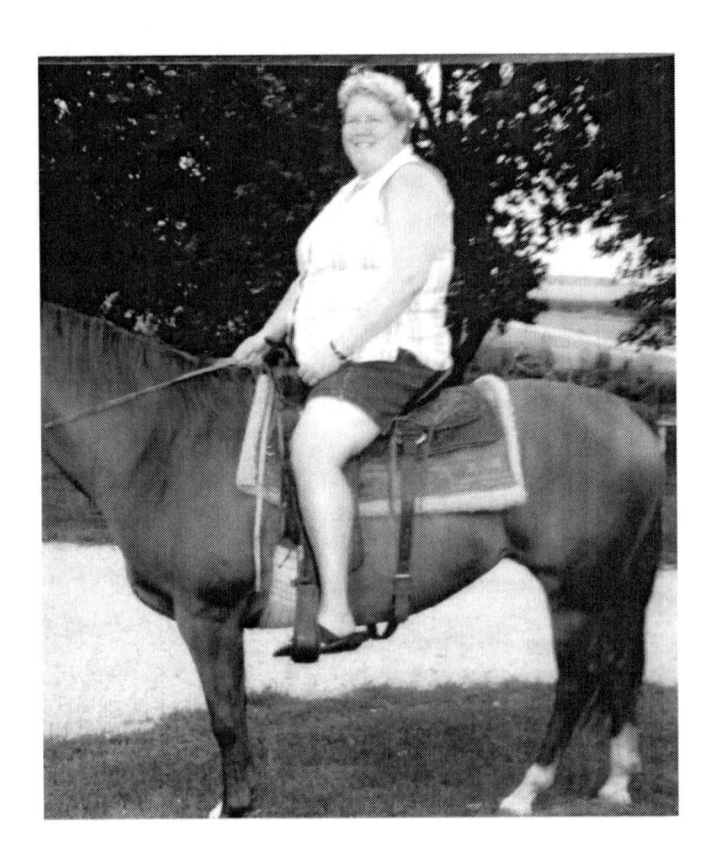

There was definitely a transition to more convenience foods at this time. And it wasn't that we just had to feed the four of us, at harvest time, there were also farm workers who also needed to be fed; which meant that there were always cakes and snacks around for the guys. So, at the age of 11, I was actually driving into town to collect the groceries and other necessities that could be found there. This change in family fortunes was, therefore, also associated with an increase in the amount and a decrease in the quality and healthiness of the food. And, of course, it was always around for me to indulge in when I was frustrated, insecure or bored.

I'm not sure that having to step up in this situation made me the helper, the mediator, the one to make it all OK, or whether it just developed my natural tendencies. But in any event, I sucked it up, did what I felt I was supposed to do and played my part in creating the new normal in our home.

It felt like a role reversal. I grew up fast. I took on responsibility and a degree of independence. I was resilient. There was something else. My mom's emotions were fragile. So, I learned not to rock the boat. I learned to smile at all costs. I learned not to express any sort of anxiety, frustration or anger. My emotions were locked away, consigned to that private, unseen part of me.

Not that there wasn't help from our community. People helped out in all sorts of ways, especially on the farm. That first summer, people helped a lot, doing all manner of farm chores. Everyone stepped up. The family grew closer. The community grew closer.

A combination of all these reasons meant that, by the time I entered the sixth grade, I was 5'10" and weighed 200 pounds. Believe me, you stand out. And because you do, you are constantly wondering what people really think of you. It makes you incredibly self-conscious. It makes you smile more and open up less. Or, in my case, not at all.

I did well in school. It came easily to me. I am a very visual person; if I can see it, or even visualize it, I understand it and can memorize it. Outside of academics, I developed and refined the role of "social butterfly," having lots of friends, helping them out, but never letting them in. Coming from a small community, many of the kids just hung out together at weekends, which I did when I wasn't helping around the farm or with household chores. I never got into trouble.

There were still many things that my mom couldn't do throughout my entire time at school. Sometimes, she would be in despair at her handicaps, and I knew she felt she was a burden to all of us, especially my dad. But, of course, she wasn't a burden -- she was my mom, and my dad's soul-mate, and we did everything we could to ensure her comfort and a normal life. Not that I ever talked about these feelings to anyone. I just kept on smiling.

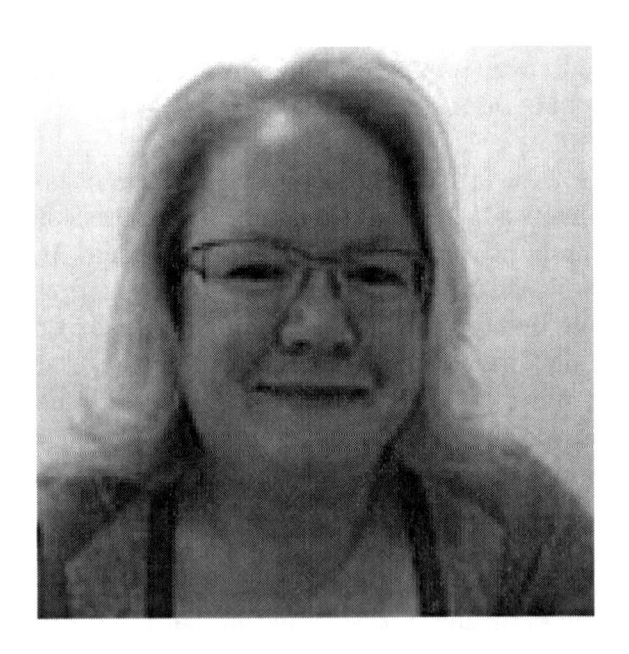

In fact, the seven years after her stroke, almost until the time I was in college, mom still had major problems. Her medications were being changed in the search of the best pharmaceutical cocktail. There was also the concern that she might have another stroke. Even worse, however, was information that she was given at the time of her hospitalization. She was told that most people with her condition don't survive more than seven years. As a result, I was on a constant vigil, waiting for any sign of her demise, through the entire time up to my high school graduation, especially my senior year -- her seventh after her initial stroke. It made me on edge whenever I thought of it -- and even when I didn't.

I continued to be active and was heavily involved in school athletics, especially in athletics where being heavy helped my involvement, like field events such as throwing the discus and putting the shot. I also played basketball, volleyball and softball.

My participation in these sports brought me into direct competition from students at other schools, who weren't always kind about my size. And it wasn't just the students at these schools, either. During one basketball game, I was pouring in the points, which prompted the opposing coach at one point to yell in frustration at his team,

"Who's guarding the fat chick?!" Just thinking about that today, makes me emotional. It's amazing that people can be so hurtful and not even know, much less care about, what they are saying and the impact they are having.

My smiling face, good grades, and athletic accomplishments actually paid off. I was awarded athletic and academic scholarships to attend Dakota State University, which was an hour away from my home in Madison, South Dakota. It was an NAIA Division III school, and I enjoyed my computer science studies as well as the sports. I enjoyed living on campus and had a lot of fun.

In my senior year in college, with the easy availability of the gym, I made my first real concerted effort at losing weight. I applied myself, mostly on the exercise side, and lost about thirty-five pounds that year. It was the first time I made a concentrated effort to lose weight focusing on exercise and using the gym.

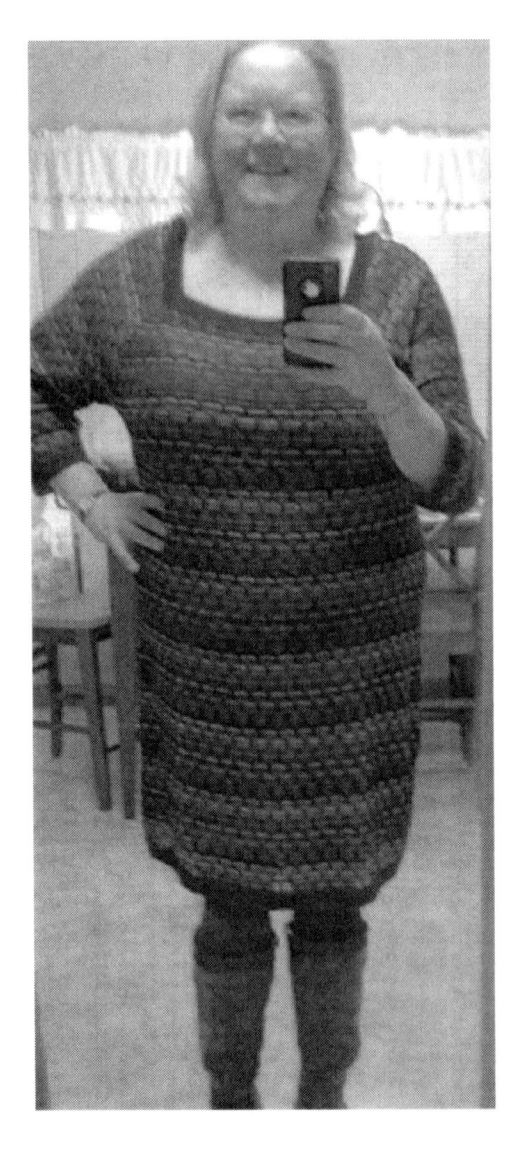

After college, I got my first job, also just an hour away from home. I was teaching and training people in software use and application. I didn't want to stray too far from home, in case I was needed. Within a year, I took a second job in Sioux Falls, also close to home. As I was establishing my career, there was part of me that felt confident and independent. But there was also another part of me that felt ugly and unattractive. I didn't want people looking at me, or judging me from the outside; please just get to know me. I didn't want to let anyone in or see me. My motto actually was, 'Die before you cry.' Nobody was going to know what was going on inside. Not even me.

For the next few years, until I was thirty, I buried my head in the sand about my weight. At my highest weight, I was 296, ninety pounds heavier than college. Around the age of thirty, I started to dabble in weight loss. I was still active, playing volleyball. I tried the Atkins diet and a variety of low-calorie plans as well as weight loss groups. I didn't do any really fad diets or take any pills. But I was still eating high processed carbs and probably eating upwards of four thousand calories a day.

In 2007, however, two significant events occurred. I was diagnosed with type II diabetes, and my grandmother passed away. This prompted another very significant development.

I had switched jobs in 2005 and my boss, Eric, was a very religious man. He was also a hugger. Initially, he would-- in the most non-threatening way-- do this to me; like putting a hand on my shoulder. I didn't like this, and told him in no uncertain terms that this was an invasion of my space.

He challenged me, lovingly. He would joke that he was going to 'convert' me. When my grandmother passed away I took the opportunity to talk to him about her faith. Where was she? Was she in Heaven? Was she a believer?

Eric chose the moment to ask me about my beliefs. What did I believe? What guides my life?

I got very emotional. Me, emotional! In front of someone else no less!

I broke down.

It just came out. I admitted I was angry at God for what had happened to my mom. But I also felt guilty for feeling angry at God.

"Don't you think that God can handle you being angry at him?" Eric responded.

I lost it. I bawled and bawled.

I had never experienced anything like that before. It was a turning point.

As it was happening, I was scared. I was actually showing my feelings, acknowledging them and letting someone observe the whole proccss.

But as I drove home that night, it was the most wonderful feeling. I was ecstatic. I felt free. I was still crying when a song came on the radio.

"God is in control," announced the lyrics. More bawling. Utter relief. It was okay to let go. I mean really let go. There was a tremendous sense of peace recognizing that I couldn't control everything -- or need to.

I was, however, into the unknown -- a whole new world. That was scary.

The next day I had questions, lots of questions. Over the course of the next few weeks, Eric, and then some of my colleagues, shared many wonderful conversations that helped me navigate this new world of emotions, of vulnerability.

Eric encouraged me to go with a co-worker and friend, a woman who was very involved with her church, to her place of worship. I was fine with that, more than fine. I wanted to learn -- really learn -- what this adventure of life was really about. As with my boss and my colleague, I found that the people at church didn't judge me. They accepted me for who I was, not who I was trying to be. And the more they did, the less I was afraid of showing them who I was; of finding out who I was. It probably took me about six months to get really comfortable with the process.

I joined a bible study group and became really integrated and still am very involved to this day.

Because of my Type II diabetes, I now became much more motivated to learn about nutrition and health in general. I became much more aware about everything I ate, limited portions and eliminated a lot of junk food. I dropped about forty-five pounds very quickly.

Not long afterwards, however, I got into a long-term relationship with a man. If I had been honest with myself, I would have realized fairly soon that it wasn't the right relationship for me. But I am a pleaser and I stayed longer than was good for me. And, as I once again sacrificed my own needs, I lost control of my eating and weight. The fact is that while I am an outgoing, passionate person, he was not. I chose the path of least resistance and stayed, sacrificing myself for perceived but illusory stability. During this time, the weight came back on, and I lost my focus on my health if not myself.

That relationship ended in 2011. That allowed me to refocus on what I really wanted to life.

Once it did, I refocused on myself and my health. I started exercising with greater regularity and for the first time, set myself specific exercise goals. When the support and encouragement of a personal trainer I decided to run my first 5k! I loved it. It gave me a true sense of accomplishment, and I wanted more. So, I am currently training for my first mini-triathlon -- a 9 mile bike ride, 2 mile run, 6 laps swim.

I was also introduced to a local nutritional weight and wellness program that focuses on eating real foods. Learning how toxic processed food really is and the huge value of clean, healthy food was a turning point for me. That's when it really clicked for me about what food really is. I started to naturally ask any time that I came into contact with food; the following question-- is this fuel or is it poison? It took six months, but I finally eliminated the processed foods, and it has made a world of difference.

I am also a member of the weight loss support group Take Off Pounds Sensibly (TOPS). The encouragement, support and accountability I have gotten from that group have made a huge difference, too. There's nothing like being around like-minded people to help you understand yourself and your habits.

I remember what my grandparents ate. The only things they bought from the store was flour and sugar, and they could have eliminated the sugar. The massive increase in the incidence of diabetes, obesity and cancer, correlates with the rise in processed foods.

My typical daily nutrition is as follows.

Breakfast is a smoothie with half an avocado, half a banana, coconut milk, ice, berries, protein powder, flaxseed, and dynamic greens.

Lunch is a salad with nuts, lean protein, complex carbs, mostly veggies.

I typically have a snack in the middle of afternoon to boost energy. This typically consists of nitrate-free deli ham, carrots, grapes, walnuts.

I cook a roast or chicken on Sunday and have that during the week with steamed or fresh vegetables. Concerned about higher sugar, I limit fruit to mornings, giving me a chance to burn off the calories.

I am sure that I was addicted to carbs, and I very rarely have any processed, high-glycemic foods. I know how difficult it is to get off them, but once you do you'll find you'll be less hungry and have a whole lot more energy.

I have a 90/10 rule which means that I'm on my plan 90% of the time and the 10% I can be "off-plan," typically something healthy. Recently, I went to a fast-food place and had a corndog. Not only did it not taste good; I was unfulfilled and hungry for the rest of the day. If you're hooked on processed carbs, work through the withdrawal, and you'll finally be able to control your appetite and the amount you eat.

There was something else that I learned when I went to the nutrition and wellness program. It's simple but hard to embrace at first. Here it is...

There's no end date.

You're not on a program that stops. You're on it forever. Once I really accepted that fact, it made it easier for me. No worrying about what's next. No worrying about maintenance. Just focusing on right now.

As I really embarked on my program fifteen months ago, one goal was to reduce, ideally eliminate, my medications. At that time, I was on four medications for my diabetes and blood pressure. Now I'm just on one-half of a pill, and I expect to be off that by the time you read this.

I had also been diagnosed with sleep apnea. My legendary energy had gotten so bad at one point that even my nephew and niece commented about it. There's no question that the obesity-apnea cycle saps your energy. Without quality sleep, your body looks for energy, typically in the form of those high-sugar carbs but all they do is ultimately zap your energy more, leaving you in a vicious cycle. Getting back to quality sleep restored my energy and thus the control I needed to take charge of my health and my life.

There was a point after I was diagnosed with diabetes that I consulted with a physician to explore the possibilities of bariatric surgery. This physician actually looked me straight in the eyes and said:

"I'm telling you as a physician that the only way you're ever going to lose weight and keep it off is the lap-band procedure. You're not going to do it any other way."

A bit like the opposing coach's "fat chick" comment, the doctor's words are indelibly imprinted in my mind. I use them often to stay motivated and to remind myself that I can do this. I am sure there are some people for whom surgery is the answer, but it's not for me. For one thing, I enjoy eating healthy foods, some of which I wouldn't be able to tolerate with surgery.

I am mature now so I can use the doctor's comments as motivation rather than sabotage. I'm sure there were times as a child when I rebelled against my mother's well-meaning comments about my eating, and as a result, they led me eat more, not less.

And what about my mom today? She is incredible. Despite the fact that some of her stroke-induced neurological problems linger to this day, and despite the fact that she is now also a breast cancer survivor, she and my dad are enjoying semi-retirement. It's fun to watch them be able to relax a bit, now, although of course, I still am the dutiful daughter who feels I need to watch out for both of them, especially since my dad is a cancer survivor, too.
I am still a teacher and a helper -- but now not at the expense of myself. I want you to know three important things.

You are not stuck. Your situation can be changed.

You are worth it.

God has a plan for you.

I feel as if I'm finally living life now. I don't feel that way because I've lost 70 pounds, I've lost the seventy pounds because I feel that way. I have a lot more self-confidence. I hope I am more honest with myself and with others. I feel much better about my body. I can hold my head up high. I'm more open to relationships. I am so much more at peace.

My experience of September 11, 2001 makes me feel I have a purpose and there's meaning in my life. God has a plan for me. I very easily could have been in the wrong place at the wrong time on September 11, but in many ways I feel as I was in the right place. It just took me a while to realize it. I have become very grateful for all my experiences and all the people in my life. I acknowledge life as a true gift and I want to cherish and make it meaningful. I have a joy for life, and I now want to share that with others.

I have changed since that conversation with my boss. In fact, rather than shrinking from hugs now, I welcome them. Instead of being the person who withdraws at the thought of an embrace, I welcome them. So much so, I even instituted Fridays as 'hug day' at my work.

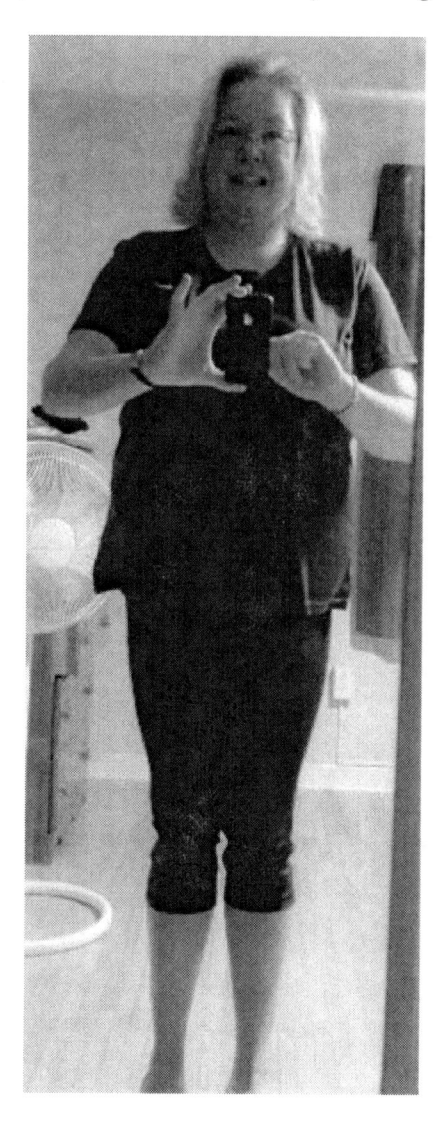

I've learned to love myself.

including international, federal, state, and local is the sole responsibility of the purchaser or reader.

Any perceived slight of any individual, group, ethnicity, race, sexual orientation, or profession is completely unintentional.

Copyright Talent Writers © 2014

CPSIA information can be obtained at www.ICGtesting.com
Printed in the USA
LVOW08s2030300315

432596LV00021B/372/P

9 781508 453567